D1404184

JUL 2 2 2011

DEADLY DISEASES AND EPIDEMICS

PNEUMONIA

DEADLY DISEASES AND EPIDEMICS

Anthrax, Second Edition

Antibiotic-Resistant Bacteria

Avian Flu

Botulism, Second Edition

Campylobacteriosis

Cervical Cancer

Chicken Pox

Cholera, Second Edition

Dengue Fever and Other Hemorrhagic Viruses

Diphtheria

Ebola and Marburg Virus, Second Edition

Encephalitis

Escherichia coli Infections, Second Edition

Gonorrhea, Second Edition

Hantavirus Pulmonary Syndrome

Helicobacter pylori

Hepatitis

Herpes

HIV/AIDS

Infectious Diseases of the Mouth

Infectious Fungi

Influenza, Second Edition

Legionnaires' Disease

Leprosy

Lung Cancer

Lyme Disease

Mad Cow Disease

Malaria, Second Edition

Meningitis, Second Edition

Mononucleosis, Second Edition

Pelvic Inflammatory Disease

Plague, Second Edition

Pneumonia

Polio, Second Edition

Prostate Cancer

Rabies

Rocky Mountain Spotted Fever

Rubella and Rubeola

Salmonella

SARS, Second Edition

Smallpox

Staphylococcus aureus Infections

Streptococcus (Group A), Second Edition

Streptococcus (Group B)

Syphilis, Second Edition

Tetanus

Toxic Shock Syndrome, Second Edition

Trypanosomiasis

Tuberculosis

Tularemia

Typhoid Fever

West Nile Virus, Second Edition

Whooping Cough

Yellow Fever

DEADLY DISEASES AND EPIDEMICS

PNEUMONIA

Christine Adamec

Consulting Editor
Hilary Babcock, M.D., M.P.H.,
Infectious Diseases Division,
Washington University School of Medicine,
Medical Director of Occupational Health (Infectious Diseases),
Barnes–Jewish Hospital and St. Louis Children's Hospital

Foreword by
David L. Heymann
World Health Organization

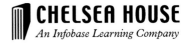

CHELSEA HOUSE
An Infobase Learning Company

Pneumonia

Chelsea House
An imprint of Infobase Learning
132 West 31st Street
New York NY 10001

Library of Congress Cataloging-in-Publication Data

Adamec, Christine A., 1949-
  Pneumonia / Christine Adamec ; consulting editor, Hilary Babcock ; foreword by David L. Heymann.
     p. cm. — (Deadly diseases and epidemics)
  Includes bibliographical references and index.
  ISBN-13: 978-1-60413-451-3 (hardcover : alk. paper)
  ISBN-10: 1-60413-451-8 (hardcover : alk. paper)   1. Pneumonia.   I. Title.
II. Series.
  RA644.P8A33 2011
  616.2'41—dc22

                                                      2011012187

Chelsea House books are available at special discounts when purchased in bulk quantities for businesses, associations, institutions, or sales promotions. Please call our Special Sales Department in New York at (212) 967-8800 or (800) 322-8755.

You can find Chelsea House on the World Wide Web at
http://www.infobaselearning.com

Text design by Terry Mallon
Cover design by Takeshi Takahashi
Composition by Newgen North America
Cover printed by Yurchak Printing, Landisville, Pa.
Book printed and bound by Yurchak Printing, Landisville, Pa.
Date printed: June 2011
Printed in the United States of America

10 9 8 7 6 5 4 3 2 1

This book is printed on acid-free paper.

All links and Web addresses were checked and verified to be correct at the time of publication. Because of the dynamic nature of the Web, some addresses and links may have changed since publication and may no longer be valid.

Table of Contents

Foreword

Communicable diseases kill and cause long-term disability. The microbial agents that cause them are dynamic, changeable, and resilient: They are responsible for more than 14 million deaths each year mainly in developing countries.

Approximately 46% of all deaths in the developing world are due to communicable diseases, and almost 90% of these deaths are from AIDS, tuberculosis, malaria, and acute diarrheal and respiratory infections of children. In addition to causing great human suffering these high-mortality communicable diseases have become major obstacles to economic development. They are a challenge to control either because of the lack of effective vaccines, or because the drugs that are used to treat them are becoming less effective because of antimicrobial drug resistance.

Millions of people, especially those who are poor and living in developing countries, are also at risk from disabling communicable diseases such as polio, leprosy, lymphatic filariasis, and onchocerciasis. In addition to human suffering and permanent disability, these communicable diseases create an economic burden—both on the workforce that handicapped persons are unable to join, and on their families and society, upon which they must often depend for economic support.

Finally, the entire world is at risk of the unexpected communicable diseases, those that are called emerging or reemerging infections. Infection is often unpredictable because risk factors for transmission are not understood, or because it often results from organisms that cross the species barrier from animals to humans. The cause is often viral, such as Ebola and Marburg hemorrhagic fevers and severe acute respiratory syndrome (SARS). In addition to causing human suffering and death, these infections place health workers at great risk and are costly to economies. Infections such as Bovine Spongiform Encephalopathy (BSE) and the associated new human variant of Creutzfeldt-Jakob disease (vCJD) in Europe, and avian influenza A (H5N1) in Asia, are reminders of the seriousness of emerging and reemerging infections. In addition, many of these infections have the potential to cause pandemics, which are a constant threat to our economies and public health security.

Science has given us vaccines and anti-infective drugs that have helped keep infectious diseases under control. Nothing demonstrates the effectiveness of vaccines better than the successful eradication of smallpox, the decrease in polio as the eradication program continues, and the decrease in measles when routine immunization programs are supplemented by mass vaccination campaigns.

Likewise, the effectiveness of anti-infective drugs is clearly demonstrated through prolonged life or better health in those infected with viral diseases such as AIDS, parasitic infections such as malaria, and bacterial infections such as tuberculosis and pneumococcal pneumonia.

But current research and development is not filling the pipeline for new anti-infective drugs as rapidly as resistance is developing, nor is vaccine development providing vaccines for some of the most common and lethal communicable diseases. At the same time, providing people with access to existing anti-infective drugs, vaccines, and goods such as condoms or bed nets—necessary for the control of communicable diseases in many developing countries—remains a great challenge.

Education, experimentation, and the discoveries that grow from them are the tools needed to combat high-mortality infectious diseases, diseases that cause disability, or emerging and reemerging infectious diseases. At the same time, partnerships between developing and industrialized countries can overcome many of the challenges of access to goods and technologies. This book may inspire its readers to set out on the path of drug and vaccine development, or on the path to discovering better public health technologies by applying our current understanding of the human genome and those of various infectious agents. Readers may likewise be inspired to help ensure wider access to those protective goods and technologies. Such inspiration, with pragmatic action, will keep us on the winning side of the struggle against communicable diseases.

David L. Heymann
Assistant Director General
Health Security and Environment
Representative of the Director General for Polio Eradication
World Health Organization
Geneva, Switzerland

1

An Overview

Jimmy, 12, heard his parents talking in hushed tones about Nana, his great-grandmother, who had just been hospitalized for pneumonia yesterday. He hoped Nana, who was in her eighties—although he couldn't remember her exact age—would get well fast, because she had promised to come watch him at the playoffs on Saturday. Jimmy knew that Nana would love to see the game, and he had already decided that he wouldn't be embarrassed when she screamed his name and waved her arms around wildly like she always did when she saw him come out to the field. But the next morning, Jimmy's parents told him sadly that Nana didn't make it—she had complications and had died, and there was nothing more that the doctors could have done for her. Jimmy was stunned—wasn't pneumonia like a really bad cold? Why didn't the doctors give Nana some extra medicine if she was that sick? He knew that Nana was old, but she was fine the last time he had seen her, just a few weeks ago. Jimmy was angry and confused, and he wanted answers.

Pneumonia is a serious lung infection and inflammation that is usually caused by a virus or bacterium, or, rarely, is caused by a fungus. Pneumonia can be mild, serious, or even fatal in its impact on the individual. According to infectious diseases medical professor Burke A. Cunha, M.D., in his 2010 book *Pneumonia Essentials*, the pathogen **Streptococcus pneumoniae** causes up to 40% of all **community-acquired pneumonia** (CAP), which are those lung infections that are usually contracted when individuals are still residing at home, in contrast to the infections that are contracted while the individual is being treated in a hospital, residing in a nursing home, or receiving major medical treatment in another type of a health care facility, such as a dialysis center.[1]

S. pneumoniae was first identified by Louis Pasteur in 1881 when he isolated the bacterium from the saliva of a child with rabies.[2] *S. pneumoniae* is a gram-positive bacterium, which means that when tested in the laboratory with a special stain, this particular bacteria will show up as blue or violet. In contrast, gram-negative bacteria show up as pink or red in a gram stain. **Gram's stains** help to identify the infecting microbe, which in turn helps to determine what antibiotic would be most effective for the patient. However, they are not always accurate. In addition, since so many people with pneumonia have *S. pneumoniae*, the doctor may simply assume it is the cause and treat with **antibiotics** effective against this pathogen, unless the individual is extremely ill and requires hospitalization and further testing.

FOUR PRIMARY CLASSES OF PNEUMONIA

There are four broad classifications of pneumonia that are used by physicians and health care experts today in the United States, including community-acquired pneumonia (CAP), **health care–associated pneumonia (HCAP)**, **hospital-acquired pneumonia (HAP)**, and **ventilator-associated pneumonia (VAP)**.[3] These general types are important to know because doctors may differentiate their diagnosis, treatment, and even the prognosis (outlook) of the patient, depending on the believed origin of the pneumonia. It is also important to know if it is an infection that was contracted 48 hours or more after the person was admitted to the hospital and thus was not already present before admission.[4] Note that some experts use the term **nosocomial** to describe all infections that develop while a patient is in a hospital.

If the infection is believed to be a HAP infection, then more diagnostic tests are generally performed than would be done if the infection was believed to be a CAP infection. The reason for this is that patients with HAP are more likely to be infected with unusual and even antibiotic-resistant pathogens compared to patients with a CAP infection. As a result, it is more important to try to isolate the type of bacterium that these patients have than with CAP patients.

Patients with a HAP infection may also require different and/or higher dosages of medications. In addition, people with CAP generally have a much better prognosis than individuals with the other forms of pneumonia, largely because people with CAP have more common bacteria that are easier to eradicate. In addition, they include a healthier population of people because they were not already in a hospital or nursing home when they developed pneumonia.

Despite these factors, however, some patients with CAP do need to be hospitalized and may become very ill.

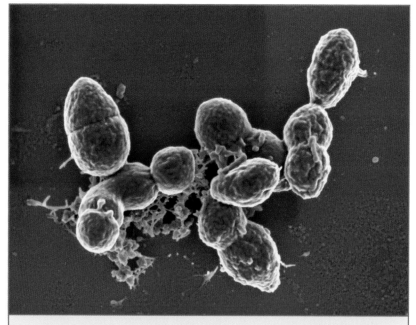

Figure 1.1 *Streptococcus pneumoniae* causes up to 40% of all community-acquired pneumonia. (© Photo Researchers)

ANTIBIOTIC-RESISTANT INFECTIONS ARE PROBLEMATIC TODAY

Infections that are resistant to antibiotics are an increasing problem around the world. In 2010, the Infectious Diseases Society of America noted in testimony to Congress that hospital-acquired antibiotic-resistant infections kill almost 100,000 people per year in the United States, and these infections cost the health care system up to $34 billion per year.[5]

Health Care–Associated Pneumonia

Health care–associated pneumonia (HCAP) is a classification that includes individuals who contracted pneumonia while they were living in nursing homes or at other long-term care facilities, as well as patients receiving kidney dialysis, or those who contracted pneumonia when they received same-day surgery.[6] This category does not, however, include people who go to regular outpatient appointments with their physicians.

Community-Acquired Pneumonia

As mentioned, CAP refers to any type of pneumonia that is contracted outside a hospital or health care setting. As a result, the individual may have contracted pneumonia while at work, at school, or when he or she was at many other sites. There are many different risk factors for CAP, and the risk is often directly related to each particular pathogen. For example, addicts who inject illegal drugs are more likely to contract CAP that is caused by the pathogens *S. aureus, M. tuberculosis,* and *S. pneumoniae.*[7]

Hospital-Acquired Pneumonia

Hospital-acquired pneumonia (HAP) is a very serious condition because the person who develops HAP was already sick

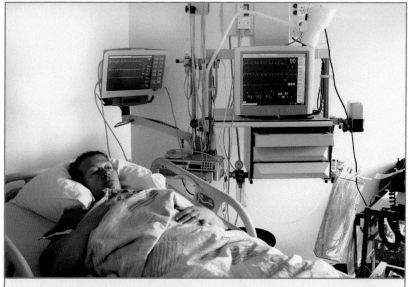

Figure 1.2 **Hospital-acquired pnemonia (© Shutterstock)**

and in the hospital for another ailment when he or she con-tracted pneumonia, and thus is usually in a weakened condi-tion compared to non-hospitalized patients with pneumonia. After urinary tract infections, pneumonia is the most common infection contracted while in the hospital.[8] It is also true that the pneumonia-causing germs that are found in a hospital envi-ronment are generally more serious and more dangerous than the pathogens that may be acquired in the community. The National Institutes of Health (NIH) says that the most common microbes affecting patients infected with HAP are *Staphylococ-cus aureus* and gram-negative bacteria.[9]

According to the NIH, individuals who are most at risk for HAP include people who fit one or more of the following risk factors:

- Those with chronic lung disease

- Elderly individuals

- Alcoholics

- Individuals who have aspirated (breathed in) material into their lungs

- Individuals with poor immune systems because of illness or disease

- Those who have had chest surgery[10]

Ventilator-Associated Pneumonia

Individuals who require the use of ventilator assistance because they cannot breathe on their own have an increased risk for developing pneumonia. These individuals are already very ill and are often receiving treatment in the intensive care unit (ICU) of the hospital. According to Antoni Torres and colleagues in their article on HAP and VAP in *Clinical Infectious Diseases*, up to 30% of the patients who need a ventilator for longer than a 48-hour period will develop VAP.[11] Factors associated with VAP include the presence of **acute respiratory distress syndrome (ARDS)**, chronic pulmonary disease, and neurological disease.

Death rates from VAP can be as high as 40%. In addition, if VAP is caused by resistant and invasive microbes, then the fatality rate may be 70% or greater.[12]

KEY SYMPTOMS AND SIGNS OF PNEUMONIA

Different types of pneumonia may have somewhat different symptoms and signs, but there are broad common indicators. (*Symptoms* are complaints of the patient, such as fatigue, while *signs* are measurable indicators of disease, such as fever or blood pressure.) It should also be noted, however, that elderly patients are less likely than patients of other ages to have common symptoms of pneumonia; instead, symptoms such as confusion are much more commonly observed in older

MANY EAR INFECTIONS ARE CAUSED BY PNEUMONIA BACTERIA

According to the Centers for Disease Control and Prevention, about a third of all cases of acute otitis media (severe middle ear infections, which are much more common in children than adults) are caused by some of the same bacteria that also cause pneumonia: *Streptococcus pneumoniae*. The CDC also notes that more than 3 million children under the age of five develop acute otitis media each year.[13]

individuals.[14] In general, many adults with pneumonia present with the following symptoms:

- Cough

- Fever

- Chills

- Sweating

- Fatigue

- Shortness of breath (**dyspnea**)

- Muscle pain

- Chest pain

- Rusty-looking **sputum**

The cough of a person with pneumonia is usually "productive," which means that the sputum, a mixture of mucus and sometimes of blood as well, is coughed up from the lungs. Sometimes doctors have the sputum analyzed to isolate the particular pathogen causing the pneumonia, and this is especially the case with hospitalized patients. However, the absence of coughing up any sputum—or even the absence of a cough—may occur sometimes with pneumonia.

The chest of the person with pneumonia may hurt because of frequent coughing as well as from very severe congestion of the lungs.

A body temperature above normal is common with pneumonia, and if the fever rises to a sustained 102°F., then the individual should consult with a physician. This fever sign is especially true among individuals who are at high risk for pneumonia, such as babies and small children, the elderly, and those individuals who are immunocompromised (those with weak immune systems).

Fever that also presents with chills is symptomatic of pneumonia. Most people do not experience chills one moment and profuse perspiration shortly thereafter unless they are very ill. Chills and sweating are common symptoms with pneumonia.

Severe tiredness is another common symptom of pneumonia, as well as with many other diseases. When accompanied with fever, cough, and other symptoms, fatigue may indicate the presence of pneumonia.

It can be hard to catch one's breath and it may even be painful to breathe when pneumonia is the underlying problem from which the individual suffers.

Myalgia (muscle aches and pains) is another common symptom of pneumonia, when accompanied by fever and other symptoms.

Children with pneumonia, especially children ages five and younger, may experience such symptoms as high fever, rapid breathing, cough, loss of appetite, and wheezing. They may also experience chills and struggle to breathe, with the chest visibly retracting during inhalation. Infants may have hypothermia (below-normal temperatures), convulsions, and a loss of consciousness.

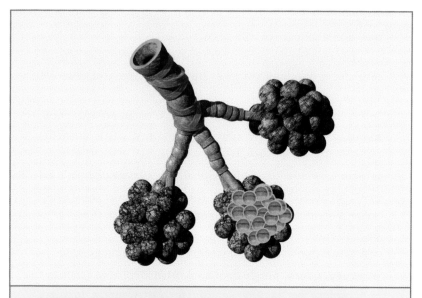

Figure 1.3 **Alveoli, microscopic air sacs in the lungs, fill with fluids as a symptom of pneumonia. (© Visuals Unlimited)**

RISK FACTORS AND PREDICTORS OF PNEUMONIA

Established risk factors for pneumonia include increased age, depressed immune system, history of smoking, and emphysema or asthma.

In a study of more than 17,000 patients of all ages in England, published in 2009 in the *British Journal of General Practice*, researcher Yana Vinogradova and colleagues found several new risk factors for pneumonia, including a greater risk for those patients who had experienced a past stroke or a transient ischemic attack (mini-stroke), as well as those patients who were diagnosed with rheumatoid arthritis, Parkinson's disease, cancer, multiple sclerosis, dementia, or osteoporosis.[15]

In an earlier study, published in 2007 in the *American Journal of Emergency Medicine*, the researchers reviewed 421 medical records of individuals with severe cough, seeking predictive factors for the diagnosis of community-acquired pneumonia. They found that an age greater than 50 years, along with abnormal vital signs such as hypoxemia (abnormally low blood levels of oxygen), fever, tachycardia (rapid heartbeat), and tachypnea (very rapid breathing) were all significant predictors for pneumonia. The researchers also found that abnormal vital signs were significantly predictive for pneumonia, regardless of the patient's age.[16]

2

Historical Background

It was 1900 and Dr. Black had done everything he could to help poor little Nellie, age six. She was extremely ill with pneumonia, and he had used a lancet this morning to bleed her again. Nellie had a high fever, was coughing severely, and was semiconscious. Dr. Black dared not bleed her again today because Nellie was so weak that he didn't know if she could survive another treatment. The doctor told her parents to prepare for the worst and pray, because it was out of his hands now. They were terribly upset because they had already lost two other children to pneumonia. Dr. Black left the family with a heavy heart. Sadly, his concern was justified. That night, Nellie died.

For thousands of years, pneumonia was the worst or one of the worst of the known diseases, particularly during periodic epidemics of **influenza**, which often led to pneumonia. Many people died of pneumonia in past years before they even had the chance to become elderly and die later of heart disease or cancer, the two most common causes of death in the United States today. Until the twentieth century, doctors did not know how to treat pneumonia effectively, nor did they have access to antibiotics, so they used age-old methods such as bleeding the patient, ostensibly to get the "bad blood" out, as well as other methods that rarely worked.

Louis Pasteur first isolated *Streptococcus pneumoniae* in 1881 but the pathogen was confused with other causes of pneumonia until the Gram's stain was developed in 1884, enabling the identification of *S. pneumoniae*.[1] In 1928, Alexander Fleming discovered the first antibiotic. This finding was a major game-changer in the historic fight against pneumonia because it provided a means to destroy many pathogens. In fact, antibiotics became so effective at treating pneumonia from the 1940s to the 1970s that many physicians and others thought that the disease was conquered for good. Unfortunately, they were wrong, and pneumonia continued to kill people every year. The first commercially available vaccine against one kind of pneumonia in the United States was developed in 1977.

TREATMENTS FOR PNEUMONIA THROUGH THE AGES

The extreme coughing and shortness of breath that characterizes pneumonia, as well as the fever and weakness that are also common with this condition, were well-known and much-feared symptoms in past years. Many physicians persisted in using the same failed methods, such as bleeding, primarily because such treatments were all that they had in their armamentarium of remedies. Doctors also treated pneumonia with a variety of substances that may sound bizarre today, such as quinine, caffeine, and cocaine, all ingredients referred to as treatments in a published discussion on the treatment of pneumonia in 1913.[2] One physician advocated high dosages of glucose for patients with pneumonia, using this treatment for years, although ultimately he gave up on it.[3]

The Alcohol Treatment

Some doctors favored giving patients with pneumonia copious quantities of alcohol, although patients were encouraged to eat as well. In 1897, S. L. Abbot, M.D., described his treatment of an 18-year-old female patient with **bronchial pneumonia** or double pneumonia (pneumonia in both lungs) who was in critical condition and refusing to take any nourishment. The doctor ordered her to take diluted French brandy, and the next morning, he found the patient had drunk about 16 ounces of the brandy.

Abbot continued this treatment for two more days and then substituted whiskey for brandy on the fourth day through the eighth day. On day eight, the patient felt better, refused any further alcohol, and began eating a light diet.[4] Why the patient survived on alcohol alone is unknown, although it is logical to assume that without her liquid refreshment, she would have died.

Some doctors prescribed alcohol to all their patients with pneumonia, while others only gave alcohol to alcoholic patients with pneumonia. Alcohol enabled patients to rest and calmed them, and was one of the few remedies available in past years. The logic behind giving alcohol to alcoholics was probably to avoid an attack of delirium tremens, a life-threatening physical reaction to the sudden withdrawal of alcohol among those individuals who are addicted to this substance.[5]

Bleeding/Bloodletting

Bloodletting, an age-old remedy and one that was prescribed for patients with pneumonia as well as those with other serious and life-threatening diseases, was used by doctors to rid the patient of "bad humors," with the hope that the remaining so-called good blood would rally and make the patient well. The patient was often bled to the point of unconsciousness. Sometimes leeches were used to extract the blood instead of lancets or other methods of causing the patient to bleed. The leeches usually fell off the patient when they were engorged with blood, but sometimes vinegar or salt was needed to force their release. In some instances as many as 100 leeches were used on a patient.[6] Some experts believe that President George Washington, who died of pneumonia, may have died prematurely because of excessive bloodletting.

According to Gilbert R. Seigworth, M.D., bloodletting was first used as a medical treatment by the ancient Egyptians. It was most popular in the early nineteenth century, but largely died out as a treatment by the end of the century, although some doctors continued to support bleeding patients as a therapy into the 1920s.[7] Doctors who used bleeding didn't realize that causing a blood loss in already-weak patients was a counterproductive treatment.

The Open-Air Treatment

In contrast with shutting up patients with pneumonia in dark rooms with all the windows tightly closed, some doctors favored the open-air treatment described by George E. Rennie, M.D., in his article published in the *British Medical Journal* in 1907.[8] Rennie believed that providing fresh air could offer more oxygen to the patient with pneumonia and could somehow "aerate" the blood of the sick patient.

According to Rennie, "My routine treatment of this disease consists in at once placing the patient on the balcony or verandah of the hospital, where they are kept night and day. A screen is placed round the head of the bed to keep the cold winds from blowing directly on the Patient."[9] Rennie claimed a high success rate, and said his open-air treatment failed for him only in the case of one man over age 60, who was nearly dead when he was admitted to the hospital. In retrospect, it is hard to understand how merely being outdoors could "cure" patients, although not being in close quarters with other sick patients may have improved the prognosis of some patients.

Crude Vaccines Used with Very Sick Patients

Some doctors in the early twentieth century tried to treat their pneumonia patients with a vaccine, but they used the vaccine on extremely ill patients, who almost invariably died. For example, Everett A. Bates, M.D., reporting his findings in 1917 in the *Boston Medical and Surgical Journal* (now the *New England Journal of Medicine*), said that he had tried a vaccine obtained from a laboratory of Tufts Medical School and "starting with enthusiasm, saw it fail in those cases where it was most needed—namely, the very sick and the fatal cases."[10]

Bates also noted that the vaccine seemed to work best in patients with a very early form of the disease—so early, in fact, that the person could not be diagnosed by most doctors. Of course, in the United States today, the pneumonia vaccine is given to people at risk for developing pneumonia, well before they contract or develop any symptoms of the disease. It is not administered to sick patients.

The Mercurochrome Treatment

Some doctors tried their own unusual remedies for pneumonia. For example, in 1925, Lewis D. Hoppe and William T. Freeman, both medical doctors, reported treating children suffering from pneumonia with an intravenous administration of Mercurochrome, a mercury-based and antibacterial substance normally used in the twentieth century to treat children's external scrapes. Before they initiated their treatment of the children, the doctors first tested their Mercurochrome therapy on rabbits, guinea pigs, and dogs that they had injected with pneumonia viruses, both to see if the treatment worked and also to determine the proper dosage to administer to the children.

According to the doctors, they treated 23 pneumonic children with intravenous Mercurochrome, and a control group of 23 children with pneumonia did not receive the Mercurochrome treatment. The doctors found that 39% of the control group children died, compared with 8.5% of the children in the Mercurochrome group. The doctors reported no apparent mercury poisoning or other effects in the surviving children who had received the Mercurochrome.[11] This treatment, however, apparently did not become a standard treatment for children with pneumonia.

Sulfonamide and penicillin were the first antibiotics used to treat pneumonia, and in later years, many other antibiotics were developed.

HISTORY OF THE PNEUMONIA VACCINE

The first crude vaccine against pneumonia for adults was developed in 1917. The original impetus for the development of a vaccine was a massive fatality rate (35%) from pneumonia among South African gold miners in 1895. There were no antibiotics available at this time. The gold mine owners sought a vaccine to help their workers and eventually enlisted Almroth

Wright, who had earlier developed a vaccine against typhoid fever.[12] Wright and others worked on the problem of developing a pneumonia vaccine, but did not find a sufficiently efficacious or side effect–free vaccine.

Finally, in 1944, the E. R. Squibb Company produced a pneumonia vaccine that was clearly effective. It was tested on airmen at the Air Force Technical Training School in South Dakota, where the population had previously suffered epidemic levels of pneumonia. The researchers found it was 90% effective and had no side effects other than temporary pain at the site where the drug was injected.[13]

By 1945, penicillin was often used to treat pneumonia among soldiers in the United States Army during World War II. However, there were some drawbacks. For example, Lieutenant Colonel J. Murray Kinsman and colleagues reported in the *Journal of the American Medical Association* that the drug was given to patients every three hours with painful intramuscular injections (since oral drugs were not available at that time). Kinsman noted that the death rate from pneumonia had decreased from 28% in World War I to less than 1% in World War II, in large part due to treatment with antibiotics.[14]

PNEUMONIA VACCINE IS TRUMPED BY ANTIBIOTICS

One trend emerged that completely overshadowed the long-awaited success of the pneumonia vaccine: the introduction of penicillin in 1944. Pencillin was viewed as a wonder drug and a godsend by most physicians as well as by the general public. Streptomycin was introduced in 1945, followed by other antibiotics used to treat pneumonia, such as chloramphenicol (1947) and chlortetracycline (1948). Physicians began to believe it silly and futile to vaccinate people against pneumonia. As a result, Squibb withdrew its pneumonia vaccine from the market in 1951, deciding nobody wanted it. The vaccine for pneumonia did not become available again until 1977.

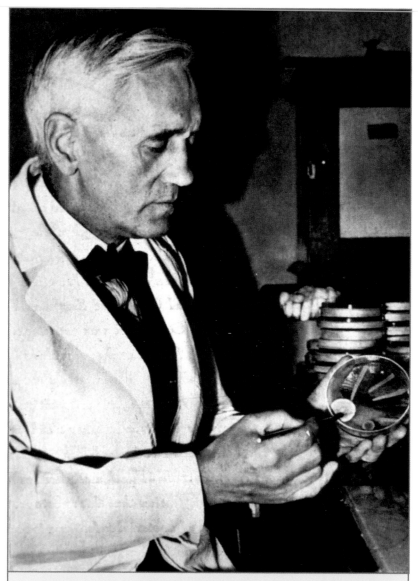

Figure 2.1 In 1928, Alexander Fleming discovered the first antibiotic. (National Library of Medicine)

Some people challenged the protocol of relying solely upon antibiotics, such as Robert Austrian, an infectious disease expert who concentrated on studying pneumonia. Austrian said that the pneumonia prevalence was unchanged from previous years and that antibiotics had not essentially wiped out the disease. In his historical medical journal article on changing attitudes toward the pneumonia vaccine, Powel Kazanjian said that Austrian's research proved that bacteremic pneumococcal pneumonia (a complication of pneumonia in which bacteria is present in the blood itself) in adults treated with penicillin or other antibiotics had a fatality rate of 17% overall. He also said that the death rate was 25% among individuals 50 years of age or older or among those with a variety of chronic systemic illnesses.

Said Kazanjian of Austrian, "He hypothesized that those who died despite antibiotic use did so because of irreversible damage that sometimes occurred very early in infection."[15] According to this theory, such individuals had experienced damage to the body that had passed beyond the point of no return, and thus the body was no longer responsive to antibiotics.

Austrian began a study in 1967 that eventually identified 14 types of pneumocci implicated in 85% of the patients diagnosed with bacteremic infections from pneumococci. He also persisted in researching and writing about the problem of pneumonia and the importance of prevention.

THE FIRST MODERN PNEUMONIA VACCINES

In 1977, the major pharmaceutical company Merck received a license to market a pneumococcus vaccine. At that time, there was still reluctance among some physicians to recommend a pneumonia vaccine to their patients. But a new threat—the discovery of an increasing number of strains of resistant microbes—was noted by the end of the 1970s. These were germs that did not respond to penicillin, erythromycin, or to antibiotics in the cephalosporin class, which were all the antibiotics available at the time. As a result, physicians began to move toward the concept of the prevention of pneumonia rather than waiting until a patient had pneumonia and then treating it with antibiotics.[16]

According to the Immunization Action Coalition, an advocacy organization that provides vaccination information for health care professionals and the public and that concentrates on promoting the use of immunizations to prevent infections, the pneumonia vaccine that was developed in 1977 was effective against 14 types of pneumococcus.[17] This vaccine was replaced in 1983 by one that was effective against 23 different types; the latter vaccine is the pneumococcal polysaccharide vaccine or PPSV23, and it is still used as of this writing.

THE GAMBIA PNEUMOCOCCAL VACCINE TRIAL

According to the National Institute of Allergy and Infectious Diseases, the government of Gambia in Africa, in concert with the British Medical Research Council, conducted a four-year study starting in 2001 to determine if the pneumococcal vaccine was truly effective at preventing pneumococcal infections in small children. The researchers vaccinated and then followed up with more than 17,000 children who were vaccinated at the ages of six to 51 weeks, comparing them to children who were given placebos.[18]

Their research confirmed that the pneumococcal vaccine was very effective, and it reduced childhood deaths by 16% among those children who received the vaccine. In addition, vaccinated children also had a 15% lower hospitalization rate than did unvaccinated children.[19]

An estimated 80% of all adults who receive PPSV23 will develop antibodies (proteins that the body generates in order to target specific infections) and these antibodies fight against the pneumococcus if they encounter them. Most people will develop these important antibodies within two to three weeks after they receive the vaccine.[20] It is also the vaccine given to adults ages 65 and older and other high-risk groups, such as children and adults with sickle-cell disease or adults who smoke.[21]

A VACCINE FOR CHILDREN

A separate pneumonia vaccine, PCV7, also known as Prevnar, was specifically created for infants and children, and was licensed for treatment in the United States in 2000. PCV7 is effective against seven major strains of pneumonia bacteria. In 2010, PCV13 (Prevnar 13) replaced PCV7 as the pneumonia vaccine used to protect infants and young children from pneumonia. It protects against 13 different strains of pneumonia bacteria.[22]

3

Biology of Pneumonia: Source of the Infection

On one otherwise routine autumn morning in the local supermarket, an elderly customer suddenly sneezed copiously on the can of peas that she was holding in the canned goods aisle. She then decided that she didn't really want them—she'd rather have carrots for dinner. So she wiped the can with her hand to get the germs off, since she knew that she had a bad cold and did not want anyone else to get it. But it wasn't enough. Most of the streptococcus germs that she had inadvertently placed on the can when she had sneezed on it were still there, ready for the next available victim.

A few minutes later, a woman, age 26, entered the same canned food aisle and she decided that canned peas would be a good vegetable for her family to eat with their dinner. So she picked up the can that the older woman had returned—and the younger woman also unknowingly received the streptococcus pathogens. Her nose itched so she scratched it, placing some of the germs on her nose and some on her mouth when she accidentally touched these body parts. Shortly thereafter, the mom picked up her three-year-old son at the day care center, transferring some active streptococcus germs to him. The boy hugged his teacher and a couple of friends good-bye, unwittingly dispersing more streptococcus germs to these other individuals. And the cycle continued on thereafter.

Not everyone who unknowingly received the germs became ill. The elderly woman become sicker a day later, and was treated for a "strep throat" by her doctor. The mother also developed a throat infection and received antibiotics. Her resilient son remained well, as did his teacher. One of the toddlers at the day care became very ill, and he was subsequently diagnosed with pneumonia. This child was hospitalized for a few days and, fortunately, made a complete recovery.

TYPES OF MICROBES THAT CAUSE PNEUMONIA

The pathogens that cause pneumonia vary depending on whether a patient is non-hospitalized (ambulatory), is hospitalized but is not in the intensive care unit (ICU), or is severely ill and receiving treatment in the ICU of the hospital. *Streptococcus pneumoniae* or other pathogens are the cause of community-acquired pneumonia (CAP).

For example, as can be seen from Table 3.1, **Legionella**, which is the pathogen that causes Legionnaires' disease, is rare among ambulatory pneumonia patients (those who are

Table 3.1   Common Etiologies of Community-Acquired Pneumonia by Severity of Illness

Ambulatory Patients	Hospitalized (non-ICU) Patients	Severe (ICU) Patients
S. pneumoniae	*S. pneumoniae*	*S. pneumoniae*
M. pneumoniae	*M. pneumoniae*	*S. aureus*
H. influenzae	*C. pneumoniae*	*Legionella spp.*
C. pneumoniae	*H. influenzae*	Gram-negative bacilli
Respiratory viruses[a]	*Legionella spp.*	*H. influenzae*
	Aspiration respiratory viruses[b]	

[a] excluding *Pneumocystis spp.*
[b] influenza A and B, adenovirus, respiratory syncytial virus, parainfluenza.

Source: Thomas M. File, Jr., "The Science of Selecting Antimicrobials for Community-Acquired Pneumonia (CAP)," *Journal of Managed Care Pharmacy* 15, no. 2, supplement (2009): S6. Reprinted with permission.

well enough to walk around and not need hospitalization). However, it is common among those patients who are hospitalized, whether they are hospitalized in the ICU of the hospital. In addition, *Staphylococcus aureus* and gram-negative bacilli are generally the causes in patients with pneumonia hospitalized in the ICU but not among those who are ambulatory or non-ICU patients.

Bacterial Causes of Pneumonia and Other Disorders

Bacteria often resemble spirals, rods, or balls when they are observed under a microscope. They are very tiny life forms; according to the National Institute of Allergy and Infectious Diseases, about 1,000 bacteria could exist on an area that is as small as a pencil eraser.[1] Bacteria aren't always bad organisms; for example, some bacteria help a person's body to digest food or to perform other functions. In addition, some foods such as yogurt are produced with the help of bacteria. Even streptococcus, as problematic as it often is for those with pneumonia, is not invariably a sickness-causing pathogen. Many people unknowingly carry streptococcus around in their lungs and throat, yet they experience no ill effects. However, an excessive amount of streptococcus can lead to a sore throat and further to pneumonia.

Viral Infections

Viruses are even smaller pathogens than are bacteria, and are composed of genetic material known as deoxyribonucleic acid (DNA) or ribonucleic acid (RNA) molecules. Often viruses are multisided, or they are shaped like a rod or a sphere. The influenza virus is the most frequent viral cause of pneumonia. Unfortunately, more than half of the patients who are hospitalized with CAP caused by a virus are treated with antibiotics, drugs that cannot treat a viral disease. Another issue is that the overuse of antibiotics, especially the repeated use of the same antibiotic, may lead to an increased resistance to these antibiotics in an individual. This means that when antibiotics are truly needed to fight off an individual's bacterial infection, they will not work well or sometimes at all.[2] Another issue is that when antibiotics are used very frequently among many people, the diseases themselves develop a resistance at a broader level and are more difficult to eradicate. Viruses cause up to 25% of CAP and often these infections are caused by more than one kind of virus or a mixture of virus and bacteria.[3]

Unlike bacteria, which sometimes are helpful or even necessary, viruses are not useful, and some are especially toxic to the body. In fact, in many cases, people who are infected with some kinds of viruses have no idea that they are infected because there are no apparent signs or symptoms. Alternatively, they may have symptoms of a "cold," such as a cough, runny nose, and sore throat. It lasts a few days and then the symptoms resolve themselves. In other cases, the virus is very dangerous, as when it causes pneumonia.

Fungal Infections

Fungi are the third means of causing pneumonia. A fungus is actually a plant, and the most commonly known fungi are yeast, mold, and mildew, although it is believed that there are thousands of different types of fungi on the earth, according to the National Institute of Allergy and Infectious Diseases. Some fungi are beneficial, such as those yeasts that are used to make cheese and bread, as well as beer. A disease caused by a fungus is referred to as mycotic.

In the United States, there are three major different types of fungi that can lead to the development of pneumonia, including *Coccidioides immitis*, which is located in southern California as well as in the desert of the Southwest; *Histoplasma*, fungi primarily found in the Mississippi and Ohio River valleys; and *Cryptococcus neoformans*,[4] not found in a particular location.

See Table 3.2 for a listing of various types of the primary pathogens that can cause pneumonia in adults and children.

Table 3.2   Pneumonia Pathogens

Bacterial	Fungal	Atypical Pathogens
Common	*Usually in normal hosts*	*Chlamydophila (Chlamydia) pneumoniae*
Streptococcus pneumoniae	*Histoplasma capsulatum*	*Legionella spp.*
Haemophilus influenzae	*Blastomyces dermatitidis*	*Mycoplasma pneumoniae*
Moraxella catarrhalis	*Coccidioides immitis*	*Coxiella burneti* (Q fever)
Oral anaerobic bacteria (aspiration):	*Actinomyces sp.*	*Chlamydophila psittaci*
Bacteroides spp.	*Usually in compromised hosts*	*Chlamydia trachomatis* (neonates only)
Fusobacterium spp.	*Cryptococcus neoformans*	*Francisella tularensis*
Peptostreptococcus spp.	*Nocardia asteroides*	*Mycobacterium tuberculosis*
Peptococcus spp.	*Sporothrix schenckii*	Nontuberculosis mycobacteria
Prevotella spp.	*Penicillium marneffei*	**Viral**
Streptococcus pyogenes	*Aspergillus sp.*	*Children*
Escherichia coli	*Zygomycetes*	Respiratory syncytial virus (RSV)
Klebsiella pneumoniae	*Pseudallescheria boydii*	Parainfluenza virus (types 1, 2, 3)
Uncommon	**Parasitic**	Adenovirus (types 1, 2, 3)
Acinetobacter baumanii	*Pneumocystis (carinii) jiroveci*	Influenza B virus
Actinomyces sp.	*Strongyloides stercoralis*	*Adults (common)*
Eikenella corrodens	*Paragonimus westermani*	Influenza A virus
Neisseria meningitidis	*Toxoplasma gondii*	Influenza B virus
Nocardia sp.		

Table 3.2   (*continued*)

Bacterial	Fungal	Atypical Pathogens
Pasteurella multocida		Adenovirus types 4 and 7 (military recruits)
Proteus spp.		**Adults (uncommon)**
Serratia marcescens		Adenovirus (types 1, 2, 3, 5)
Pseudomonas aeruginosa		Varicella-zoster virus (VZV)
Pseudomonas pseudomallei		Cytomegalovirus (CMV)
Yersinia pestis		Herpes simples virus (HSV-1)
Staphylococcus aureus		Respiratory syncytial virus (RSV)
		Parainfluenza virus
		Measles virus
		Avian influenza (H5N1)
		Hantavirus (HPS)
		Severe acute respiratory syndrome (SARS)

Source: Burke A. Cunha, *Pneumonia Essentials,* 3d ed. Boston: Jones and Bartlett Learning, 2010. Sudbury, MA. www.jblearning.com, p. 8. Reprinted with permission.

TRANSMISSION OF PNEUMONIA-CAUSING MICROBES

The microbes that cause pneumonia are transmitted in different ways, depending on the type of pathogen. Some microbes are aerosolized—they are transmitted in the air and they are so tiny that they are unseen and thus cannot be avoided. Microbes can also be transmitted by touching an object that an infected person has touched. This is why day care centers often have outbreaks of sick children, because small children touch many objects within the day care center and they also touch one another very frequently. It is also why items in the day care center are (or should be) regularly cleaned and why children and staff are usually urged to wash their hands frequently, especially after changing diapers or helping small children who are using the toilet.

Community-acquired pneumonia (CAP) is a common disease among children, and the annual incidence is about 40 cases per 1,000 children in North America. Children ages three weeks and older with bacterial pneumonia are most frequently infected with *Streptococcus pneumoniae*. However, most preschool children with pneumonia are infected with viruses. In addition, up to 50% of children diagnosed with CAP have mixed infections, such as a combination of *Streptococcus pneumoniae* and a viral infection, or *Streptococus pneumoniae* and *Mycoplasma pneumoniae*.[5]

Sometimes microbes are transmitted by close contact with a sick person, such as by kissing the person or having intimate sexual relations. Other forms, such as *Legionella*, are transmitted in contaminated water.

CONSIDERING MAJOR
PNEUMONIA-CAUSING PATHOGENS

As seen on Table 3.2, many types of pathogens can cause the lung infection that is known as pneumonia. However, several forms predominate, including *Streptococcus pneumoniae*, *Haemophilus influenzae*, *Mycoplasma pneumoniae*, *Chlamydophila* (formerly known as *Chlamydia*) *pneumoniae*, and *Legionella*. These five pneumonia-causing culprits are described here.

Streptococcus Pneumoniae

The most common cause of CAP, *S. pneumoniae* is a bacterium that is present in the back of the nose and throat of many children and adults throughout the United States.[6] This pathogen can spread further, into the ear, causing ear infections, or to the sinuses, causing sinus infections. If the infection spreads to the lungs, then it can cause pneumonia. According to the Centers for Disease Control and Prevention (CDC), the following individuals have the greatest risk for an infection with *S. pneumoniae*:

- Children younger than age two

- Elderly individuals ages 65 and older

- American Indians and Alaska Natives

- Children who attend group day care centers

- Individuals with compromised immune systems, such as those with **human immunodeficiency virus** (HIV) or sickle-cell disease

S. pneumoniae can also sometimes travel to the blood, causing **bacteremia**, or rarely, it could even travel to the brain, causing meningitis.

Some strains of *S. pneumoniae* are resistant to antibiotics, which is a condition referred to as *treatment resistance*. In such cases, different antibiotics or higher dosages of antibiotics may be needed, as well as hospitalization.

Haemophilus Influenzae

Haemophilus influenza, also known as the flu, is considered to be either the second or third most common cause of CAP. Individuals who are infected with this pathogen are often elderly and they may have a history of chronic lung disease. *H. influenzae* is a common presence in the oral cavity and throat tract of healthy individuals, and does not lead to pneumonia in most cases.[7]

Mycoplasma Pneumoniae

Another bacterium that may lead to the development of pneumonia is *Mycoplasma pneumoniae*, which is the smallest self-duplicating organism.[8] According to the CDC, each year an

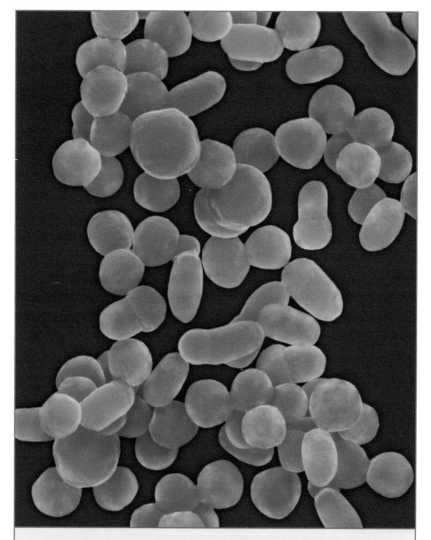

Figure 3.1 *Haemophilus influenzae*, also known as the flu, is considered to be either the second or third most common cause of CAP. (© Visuals Unlimited)

estimated 100,000 people are hospitalized with pneumonia that is caused by *M. pneumoniae* each year.[9] Both the lower and upper respiratory systems can be infected with *M. pneumoniae*.[10]

The primary symptom that is caused by this pathogen is a persistent cough, and other symptoms may also include fever, headaches, and fatigue. *M. pneumoniae* is difficult to diagnose because there are few standard tests for its detection.

Outbreaks of *M. pneumoniae* are most commonly found in crowded institutions that are occupied by adults, such as college dormitories or military settings.[11] General laboratory tests ordered by most doctors can be misleading with this pathogen; for example, with *M. pneumoniae*, the white blood cell count often shows as normal. (White blood cells fight against

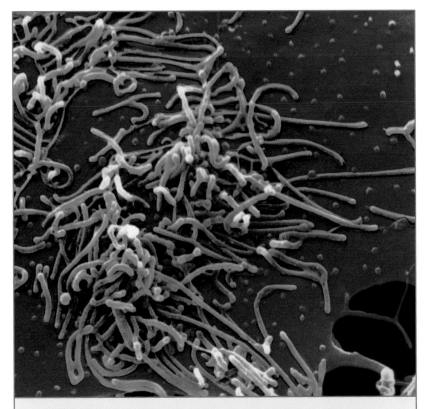

Figure 3.2 **According to the CDC, an estimated 100,000 people are hospitalized each year with pneumonia that is caused by** *M. pneumoniae*. **(© Visuals Unlimited)**

infections, and usually when there is an infection, the white blood cell count is elevated.)

M. pneumoniae is usually treated with such antibiotics as doxycycline, azithromycin, or clarithromycin, as well as with drugs such as levofloxacin (Levaquin).[12]

Chlamydophila Pneumoniae

Up to 10% of all cases of CAP worldwide are caused by *Chlamydophila pneumoniae*.[13] The incubation period (the period in which the microbes are present but before symptoms appear) is about 21 days with this pathogen.[14] Among the elderly, *Chlamydophila* pneumonia is estimated to cause up to 28% of pneumonia cases in this age group.[15]

According to the CDC, *C. pneumoniae* is transmitted from person to person in respiratory secretions. This pathogen was first isolated in a Taiwanese child in 1965.[16] *C. pneumoniae* has been theorized to be a cause of asthma in both children and adults.[17]

Headache is a more common symptom with *C. pneumoniae* than with *S. pneumoniae*. Even with treatment with the appropriate antibiotics, a cough and overall fatigue may

ASPIRATION PNEUMONIA

Most forms of pneumonia are caused by inhaled pathogens, but in some cases, saliva, food, liquids, or vomit is accidentally inhaled into the lungs, causing a condition known as aspiration pneumonia. This may occur because of a problem with swallowing or it may happen when an individual abuses alcohol or drugs and aspirates material. Aspiration pneumonia can further lead to the formation of pus in the lungs, also called a lung abscess.

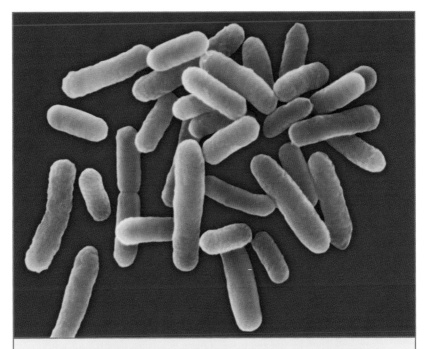

Figure 3.3 *Legionella pneumophila* may cause at least 25,000 cases of pneumonia per year in the United States, but this may be a serious underestimate, since the bacterium is difficult to isolate. (© Visuals Unlimited)

last for months in the individual who is infected with *C. pneumoniae*. In general, such drugs as tetracycline, erythromycin, or doxycycline are effective treatments for adults infected with this pathogen. Only erythromycin is used with children younger than age 8 years who are infected with *C. pneumoniae* because tetracycline and doxycycline are not recommended for treating pneumonia in younger children.

Legionella Pneumophila

Legionella is another cause of pneumonia. Its name is derived from an outbreak of disease and death that occurred in 1976 among individuals (Legionnaires) who were military veterans attending an annual convention of the American Legion in Philadelphia. Twenty-nine of the 180 attendees died.[18] This pathogen existed before the outbreak at the American Legion convention but it had not been previously identified. It was ultimately isolated from water in the air-conditioning system of the hotel convention site. *Legionella pneumophila* may cause at least 25,000 cases of pneumonia per year in the United States, but this may be a serious underestimate, since the bacterium is difficult to isolate.[19]

Individuals most in danger from *Legionella* include male smokers ages 60 and older and those with compromised immune systems. Such infected individuals are at risk for death.[20] Elderly people who have been treated with long-term corticosteroids may also be at risk for infection with *L. pneumophila*.[21]

According to the CDC, up to 18,000 individuals are hospitalized with Legionnaires' disease each year in the United States. Symptoms usually appear within two to fourteen days after exposure to the bacteria. There is a high death rate with this pathogen: Up to 30% of individuals who are infected by *Legionella* may die. Legionnaires' disease may also cause kidney failure and heart disease.

Symptoms that may occur early in the disease include confusion, cough, nausea and vomiting, diarrhea, and lethargy.

In 2007, two very ill hospitalized patients were subsequently diagnosed with Legionnaires' disease, and an investigation ultimately traced the source of the infections to a decorative water fountain (not a drinking fountain) in the hospital. Both infected patients were severely ill before they became infected with *Legionella* and each of them recalled being close to the fountain at some time before they developed pneumonia. No other individuals were found to be infected with *Legionella*.

The authors who described these patients stated that such fountains can present an unacceptable risk to those hospitals caring for immunocompromised patients—which essentially indicates all hospitals, since virtually all hospitals have at least some patients with HIV, immunocompromised patients being treated for cancer, or patients receiving dialysis, or other patients who simply have poor immune systems.[22]

In general, *Legionella* may be identified in water that is found in such sites as whirlpool baths, drinking fountains, ice machines, air-conditioning condensers, water heaters, showerheads, and other sources of water. The pathogen can be identified with the use of immunofluorescent stains.

The key symptoms and signs of Legionnaires' disease include chest pain, headache, joint pain, coughing up blood, fever, diarrhea, and lack of coordination.[23]

Individuals who are at the highest risk for contracting Legionnaires' disease are those who are immunocompromised as well as individuals who are older than 40, alcoholics, and smokers.[24]

4

Pneumonia Epidemiology

Alan, age 44, was a heavy drinker, although he did not regard himself as an alcoholic since he "only" drank four or five shots of bourbon each evening, falling asleep in his easy chair nearly every night. He was also a heavy smoker, smoking several packs of cigarettes each day. Alan was overweight and his doctor told him that he was very close to a type 2 diabetes diagnosis, and should watch what he ate and drank. But Alan figured that he was okay, since he wasn't actually diabetic yet. When his grandchild came over with a severe cold, Alan enjoyed seeing the baby. But a few days later, Alan developed a severe sore throat. Within a week, Alan could barely speak and he felt terrible, and the other guys on the assembly line demanded that Alan go to a doctor because they didn't want to get whatever he had. Alan did go to the doctor, who diagnosed him with pneumonia, putting him in the hospital. Because he was severely malnourished, the doctors treated him with vitamin supplements as well as antibiotics. But Alan kept getting worse and the doctors told him that he had nearly died. After his release from the hospital, Alan swore he'd give up booze and cigarettes, which he did, for about a week. Then the old addictions kicked in again.

Pneumonia hits many people hard, and age clearly has an impact, as do other factors. On one hand, pneumonia can seriously affect newborns and infants. At the other end of the age scale, the elderly are at high risk for pneumonia. Those with weakened immune systems are at high risk for contracting pneumonia—such as individuals who have acquired immunodeficiency syndrome (AIDS) from the human immunodeficiency virus (HIV), common variable immunodeficiency syndrome (CVID), or those who have had an organ transplant and are taking immu-nosuppressive drugs.

Other risk factors for the development of pneumonia are smoking, alcoholism, and a diagnosis of asthma. In addition, individuals with some diseases or other medical problems, such as diabetes, anemia, or a recent hip fracture, have a greater risk for pneumonia and may also have a worse prognosis than others. Of course anyone can develop pneumonia, but the risks for a severe case of the disease are much higher for individuals who fit into one or more risk categories.

MAJOR RISK FACTORS FOR DEVELOPING PNEUMONIA

Some people have an elevated risk for contracting pneumonia, according to the National Institute of Allergy and Infectious Diseases. People who fit one or more of the following categories have an increased risk:

- Are age 65 or older

- Are infected with HIV or have AIDS

- Have leukemia or lymphoma

- Receive long-term treatment with steroids

- Have kidney failure

- Have a damaged spleen or no spleen

- Receive radiation or chemotherapy for cancer

- Have an organ or bone marrow transplant[1]

WHEN AGE IS THE KEY FACTOR

Among the elderly, community-acquired pneumonia (CAP) is the number-one infectious cause of death.[2] In addition, the older the elderly person is, the greater the risk for CAP. For example, one study found that the rate of CAP was 18.2 cases per 1,000 people ages 65 to 69, but the rate leaped to 52.3 per 1,000 people in individuals ages 85 and older.[3]

Elderly people have an elevated risk for developing pneumonia for a variety of reasons. For example, individuals ages 65 and older often have more than one illness, and they may have multiple serious diseases such as diabetes, arthritis, and hypertension. They may also be taking medications that act as immunosuppressants, such as methotrexate, a drug that is given to treat rheumatoid arthritis—an autoimmune disorder—by suppressing the body's attack on itself.

Older people have a weaker immune system than when they were young and are often sedentary, which weakens the body. They may also have poor diets and have nutritional deficiencies. Older people may live in close quarters with others, as is the

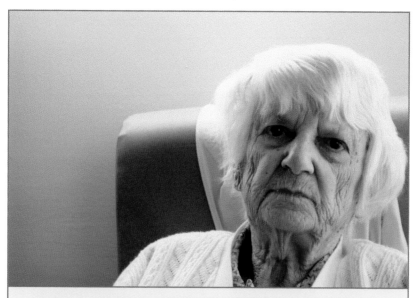

Figure 4.1 People over 65 and those living in nursing homes are at increased risk for pneumonia. (© Shutterstock)

case with older people who live in nursing homes. The risk for pneumonia increases when people live closely together, not only in nursing homes but also in dormitories or military barracks.

Premature infants, newborns, and young babies have an elevated risk for developing pneumonia because of their evolving immune systems. This is particularly true for premature infants, who have not had the chance to develop their lungs and bodies as well as a child who was born either at or close to term. In addition, premature infants are fragile beings who are fighting for their very lives usually with the assistance of neonatal intensive care units located in many hospitals. Because of their weakness, they are vulnerable to infections and to the development of pneumonia.

See Table 4.1 for more information on risk factors for CAP and also the commonly encountered pathogens among individuals with CAP. For example, alcoholism is a risk factor for *Streptococcus pneumoniae* as well as other pathogens, as seen in the table.

THE IMMUNOCOMPROMISED AND PNEUMONIA
Age is not the only factor that can increase the risk for the development of an infection with pneumonia. For example, individuals who are younger than 65 may have a problem with their immune systems, either because of medications that they take or because of immune system disorders. Some immune system disorders are acquired, as with HIV, which eventually leads to AIDS. In contrast, CVID is a genetic disorder that impairs the immune system.

THOSE WHO TAKE IMMUNOSUPPRESSANT DRUGS
Some people must take medications that impair their immune system in order to protect themselves from other medical problems, such as people who have had organ transplants; they take immunosuppressant drugs so that their immune systems

Table 4.1   Epidemiologic Conditions and/or Risk Factors Related to Specific Pathogens in Community-Acquired Pneumonia (CAP)

Condition	Commonly Acquired Pathogen(s)
Alcoholism	*Streptococcus pneumoniae*, oral anaerobes, *Klebsiella pneumoniae*, *Acinetobacter* species, *Mycobacterium tuberculosis*
Chronic obstructive pulmonary disease (COPD) and/or smoking	*Haemophilus influenzae*, *Pseudomonas aeruginosa*, *Legionella* species, *S. pneumoniae*, *Moraxella cararrhalis*, *Chlamydophila pneumoniae*
Aspiration	Gram-negative enteric pathogens, oral anaerobes
Lung abscess	CA-MRSA*, oral anaerobes, endemic fungal pneumonia, *M. tuberculosis*, atypical mycobacteria
Exposure to bat or bird droppings	*Histoplasma capsulatum*
Exposure to birds	*Chlamydophila psittaci* (if poultry: avian influenza)
Exposure to rabbits	*Francisella tularensis*
Exposure to farm animals or parturient [about to give birth] cats	*Coxiella burnetii* (Q fever)
HIV infection (early)	*S. pneumoniae, H. influenzae, M. tuberculosis*
HIV infection (late)	The pathogens listed for early infection, plus *Pneumocystis jirovecii, Cryptococcus, Histoplasma, Aspergillus* atypical mycobacteria (especially *Mycobacterium kansasii*), *P. aeruginosa, H. influenzae*
Hotel or cruise ship stay in previous two weeks	*Legionella* species
Travel to or residence in southwestern United States	*Coccidioides* species, *Hantavirus*
Travel to or residence in Southeast and East Asia	*Burkholderia pseudomallei*, avian influenza, SARS*
Influenza active in community	Influenza, *S. pneumoniae, Staphylococcus aureus, H. influenzae*
Cough more than two weeks with whoop or posttussive vomiting	*Bordetella pertussis*

Table 4.1   (*continued*)

Condition	Commonly Acquired Pathogen(s)
Structural lung disease (e.g., bronchiectasis)	*Pseudomonas aeruginosa, Burkholderia cepacia, S. aureus*
Injection drug use	*S. aureus*, anaerobes, *M. tuberculosis, S. pneumoniae*
Endobronchial obstruction	Anaerobes, *S. pneumoniae, H. influenzae, S. aureus*
In context of bioterrorism	*Bacillus anthracis* (anthrax), *Yersinia pestis* (plague), *Francisella tularensis* (tularemia)

*Note: CA-MRSA is community-acquired methicillin-resistant *Staphylococcus aureus*; SARS is severe acute respiratory syndrome.

Source: Lionel A. Mandell, et al., "Infectious Diseases Society of America/American Thoracic Society Consensus Guidelines on the Management of Community-Acquired Pneumonia in Adults," *Clinical Infectious Diseases* 44, supplement 2 (2007): p. S46. Copyright 2007 by University of Chicago Press – Journals. Reproduced with permission of University of Chicago Press – Journals in the format Tradebook via Copyright Clearance Center.

will not reject the kidney or other donated organ. Others have diseases in which the immune system attacks the body and breaks down the tissue, as with those individuals who suffer from rheumatoid arthritis. They take medications that decrease the effect of the immune system so that their pain and other symptoms are reduced.

In addition, individuals with cancer may be taking immunosuppressive medications, such as chemotherapy, and consequently be at risk for developing pneumonia. Immuno-suppressive drugs help to prevent the immune system from attacking itself, but at the same time, the weakening of the immune system caused by them leaves the individual at risk to germs that he or she could normally fight off. Chemotherapy, which kills white blood cells as well as cancer cells, is often debilitating, and can severely weaken the immune system.

THOSE WHOSE IMMUNE SYSTEMS ARE WEAKENED OR NOT WORKING: HIV, AIDS, AND COMMON VARIABLE IMMUNE DEFICIENCY

HIV is a virus transmitted through sexual contact or the use of shared needles among illegal drug users. AIDS is an advanced form of this disease, when the virus has destroyed much of the person's immune system. Individuals with HIV and AIDS are at high risk for pneumonia.

There are other immune disorders that increase the individual's risk for contracting pneumonia. For example, CVID is a genetic disorder that causes a decreased level of the immune system cells and increases the risk for upper respiratory diseases such as bronchitis and pneumonia. Often the specific genes that are implicated are unknown. The severity of the disorder varies considerably, which is why is it known as "variable" immune deficiency. CVID can be diagnosed in individuals at any age, but it is often diagnosed in young adulthood after the individual has experienced frequent hospitalizations for pneumonia. According to the National Institutes of Health (NIH), CVID may affect 1 in 25,000 people.[4]

If one person in a family has CVID, then other family members with frequent infections may be at risk as well and should be tested for CVID. Treatment may be with infusions of gamma globulin or with antibodies that will help the patient fight off infections.

THOSE WHO ARE WEAK FOR OTHER REASONS

There are other people with immune system issues who are at risk for pneumonia but are not taking immunosuppressant medications, nor do they have a disease that causes them to have a weakened immune system. Their immune systems may be weak because of a recent severe illness (such as pneumonia), a chronic and serious lack of sleep, extreme stress, poor nutrition, or other reasons. Once an individual is in a weakened state, the pathogens leading to pneumonia can move in and

WORLDWIDE PNEUMONIA IN CHILDREN IS A MAJOR PROBLEM

According to the World Health Organization (WHO), pneumonia kills 2 million children each year around the globe, and it is an infection whose effects are greater than are found with the combined worldwide effects of malaria, AIDS, and measles in

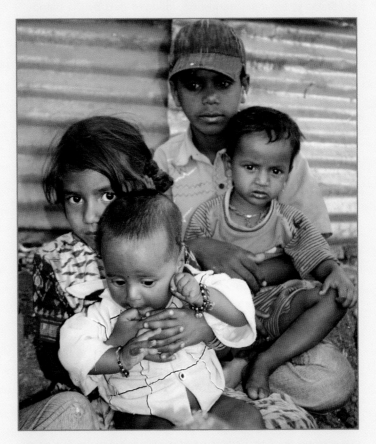

Figure 4.2 Worldwide, pneumonia each year kills more than 1.5 million children younger than 5 years of age, reports the Centers for Disease Control and Prevention. (© Shutterstock)

(continued)

children. In some parts of the world, such as in South Asia and sub-Saharan Africa, 21% of the deaths of all children are caused by pneumonia.

Streptococcus pneumoniae is the number-one cause of childhood pneumonia worldwide, followed next by the pathogen *Haemophilis influenzae*. Bacterial pneumonia is treated with antibiotics such as amoxicillin but caregivers in many countries may not recognize the symptoms or may not have access to medications. WHO says that only about half of all children with pneumonia from developing countries are taken to a health care provider.[5]

strike. Such a person might normally be able to fight off these pathogens or might in the past have developed a lesser problem than pneumonia, such as an ear infection or a "strep throat."

SOCIOECONOMIC STATUS, RACE, AND PNEUMONIA

In general, individuals who are either at or below the poverty level have a greater risk for developing pneumonia than are those who have a higher socioeconomic status. This may be because poor people generally have less access to health care, can't afford to take good care of themselves, have a restricted diet and tend to live in close quarters with others.

In the United States, American Indians and African Americans tend to have a greater risk for developing pneumonia than individuals of other races. This may be related to the fact that individuals who are American Indian or black also have a greater risk for diabetes, which is another risk factor for pneumonia, as discussed in the next section. It may also be linked to a lower socioeconomic status and a lower probability of receiving immunizations against the flu and pneumonia.

INDIVIDUALS WITH SPECIFIC MEDICAL PROBLEMS

People with diabetes have a greater risk for pneumonia than others, as do elderly individuals with hip fractures. Other medical factors and conditions can increase the risk for pneumonia as well as the risk for death. In a study of 195 elderly nursing home residents who had experienced hip fractures, those who

CONSIDERING PNEUMONIA PATIENTS ADMITTED WITH HYPOGLYCEMIA

Doctors and other research analysts frequently look for detectable patterns to help them identify particular patients who need certain treatments and medications for pneumonia and other disorders. They also look for patterns of vulnerabilities, so that they can especially watch out for these types of patients.

A study by John-Michael Gamble and colleagues, published in a 2010 issue of the *American Journal of Medicine*, found that 54 patients admitted to the hospital for pneumonia from 2000 to 2002 also had hypoglycemia (low blood sugar). These patients had an increased death rate compared to 902 pneumonia patients with normal glucose levels. This death risk persisted for up to a year after the hospitalization. The doctors noted that hypoglycemia is easily measurable and these patients may need more intensive care while in the hospital as well as subsequent to their discharge.[6]

subsequently developed pneumonia after the fracture had a 70% greater risk of death than those hip fracture patients who did not develop pneumonia, based on a study reported in 2009. The increased risk of pneumonia after hip fracture is probably due to immobilization and not being upright and fully expanding their lungs well. More than 55% of 195 subjects in the study were rehospitalized within eight weeks. The authors considered pneumonia to be a modifiable risk factor that could be prevented.[7]

Diabetes was shown to elevate the risk for developing pneumonia in a 2010 study published by Samantha F. Ehrlich and colleagues in *Diabetes Care*. The researchers analyzed medical records from 77,637 individuals with diabetes (including both type 1 and type 2 diabetes) and also records from 1,733,591 individuals without diabetes. They found that people diagnosed with diabetes also had an elevated risk for asthma and chronic obstructive pulmonary disease (COPD). The risk for pneumonia also increased with a rising hemoglobin A1C, a test that measures the blood sugar levels over a three-month period.[8] It seems logical to assume that with better blood sugar control among diabetics, the risk for developing pneumonia will decrease.

Individuals being treated for acid reflux in hospital settings have also shown an increased risk for developing HAP. In a study of 63,878 admissions to the hospital, published in the *Journal of the American Medical Association* in 2009, researchers reported that acid suppressive medications such as a proton pump inhibitor drug or a histamine 2 receptor antagonist were given to 52% of those admitted to the hospital. The researchers found that the use of proton pump inhibitors was significantly correlated with an increased risk for the patients developing HAP. The risk for the development of pneumonia was greatest in the first week of admission to the hospital.

The researchers speculated that acid suppressive medications may alter gastrointestinal and hence respiratory flora (bacteria), making it less acidic and thus more vulnerable to pathogens causing pneumonia. Further analysis is needed, but it seems logical to assume that physicians should consider carefully whether proton pump inhibitors are truly needed among patients newly admitted to the hospital.[9]

5

Complications from Pneumonia

Amy, age six, came home from the hospital today and the most important thing for her parents was that she came home at all. She had been a very active little girl before becoming sick; for example, she was on a gymnastics team. Amy suffered a severe case of pneumonia that stopped the oxygen flow to her legs. In fact, it was so bad that the infection led to the amputation of her legs in order to save her life. According to the doctors, Amy suffered from Streptococcus pneumoniae **sepsis**, *a very rare form of bacterial pneumonia with associated bloodstream infection that has a survival rate of around 10%.*

In Amy's case, the doctors did not think that she would survive. But they did their best to make it happen. The doctors put Amy into a coma for four days to try to keep her alive and she clung to life. She still needed plenty of care, however, and Amy was in the hospital for five months before she could go home. Amy had to learn how to cope without the use of her legs, and her family had to learn how to help her. No one knows why or how Amy developed this infection that cost her limbs.

Pneumonia itself is a distressing and dangerous disease for many people, but sometimes people with pneumonia develop further complications of the disease as well as exacerbations of preexisting serious conditions, such as diabetes, heart disease, or other diseases. In addition, many people suffer for at least a few weeks from the aftereffects of pneumonia; they tire very easily and may be generally more confused than usual, especially the very elderly.

Common complications of pneumonia can include the following:

- Bacteremia (bacteria in the blood)

- Lung abscess (a pus-filled area within the lung)

- Acute respiratory distress syndrome (ARDS)

- **Empyema** (a pus-filled fluid outside the lung)

- Death

BACTEREMIA

Bacteremic pneumonia is a complication of pneumonia in which bacteria are present in the blood. The pathogen can often be cultured and identified. According to the CDC, there are more than 50,000 cases of pneumococcal bacteremia that occur in the United States each year, with higher rates occurring among very young infants and the elderly. The National Institute of Allergy and Infectious Diseases reports that about 30% of individuals who have pneumococcal pneumonia will develop bacteremia.[1]

Bacteremia is dangerous because it can further escalate to a potentially fatal condition known as *sepsis*, when the body has a life-threatening and severe inflammatory response to bacteremia. The fatality rate of those with sepsis is about 20%, but among the elderly, it can be as high at 60%.[2]

Normally when individuals are infected by bacteria, their white blood cell count goes up, indicating that the immune system is fighting off an infection. If the particular pathogen is also present and identifiable in the bloodstream, this indicates a serious and potentially escalating problem. Some individuals have a higher risk for bacteremic pneumonia, such as the elderly, Native Americans, African Americans, those who smoke, and individuals with asthma, diabetes, or cancer.[3]

In a study published in the *American Journal of Public Health* on the incidence of bacteremic pneumonia by race/

Table 5.1 Incidence of Bacteremic Pneumonia in Adults According to Race/Ethnicity, Age, and Proportion of Residents Living in Poverty: United States, 2003–2004

Race/Ethnicity by Age	Population Count	No. of Cases	Incidence of Bacteremic Pneumonia per 100,000 People				
			<5% Poverty	5%–9.9% Poverty	10%–19.9% Poverty	≥20% Poverty	Overall
Total adult population	17,890,259	4,524	9.4	11.1	14.1	26.2	12.6
White, non-Hispanic	13,738,841	2,767	8.5	9.9	12.0	17.8	10.1
Black, non-Hispanic	2,353,745	1,140	12.7	14.4	20.8	37.7	24.2
Hispanic	1,031,320	148	5.9	5.6	6.1	11.2	7.2
Adults, aged 18–34 years	5,795,245	341	1.9	2.5	3.0	5.9	2.9
White, non-Hispanic	3,970,653	141	1.6	1.9	1.9	2.2	1.8
Black, non-Hispanic	929,317	142	2.6	5.0	7.5	11.4	7.6
Hispanic	572,531	31	4.3	2.6	1.4	3.8	2.7
Adults, aged 35–49 years	5,858,541	1,061	3.9	6.6	10.6	39.6	9.1
White, non-Hispanic	4,523,687	439	3.1	5.3	6.4	18.0	4.9
Black, non-Hispanic	804,471	487	13.4	14.8	21.2	58.1	30.3

Hispanic	291,768	45	0.8	3.5	9.9	16.2	7.7
Adults, aged 50–64 years	3,535,963	1,152	10.6	13.4	20.3	47.3	16.3
White, non-Hispanic	2,902,523	684	9.2	11.2	14.6	37.5	11.8
Black, non-Hispanic	390,922	315	22.2	24.5	36.8	58.7	40.3
Hispanic	114,049	31	10.3	12.4	11.8	19.9	13.6
Adults, aged, 65–79 years	1,960,136	1,027	24.5	23.0	30.2	34.7	26.2
White, non-Hispanic	1,678,195	759	21.9	19.3	26.8	34.8	22.6
Black, non-Hispanic	177,412	114	24.8	27.9	36.3	32.6	32.1
Hispanic	42,494	29	19.1	35.5	27.8	50.8	34.1
Adults, aged ≥80 years	740,374	943	69.2	61.1	61.4	59.8	63.7
White, non-Hispanic	663,783	744	62.7	53.5	50.3	55.2	56.0
Black, non-Hispanic	51,623	82	105.7	84.1	114.9	55.8	79.4
Hispanic	10,478	12	141.3	16.7	62.2	40.1	57.3

Source: Deron C. Burton, et al., "Socioeconomic and Racial/Ethnic Disparities in the Incidence of Bacteremic Pneumonia Among U.S. Adults." *American Journal of Public Health* 100, no. 10 (2010): p. 1,906. Printed with permission.

ethnicity, age, and also by the proportion of residents living in poverty, there were 4,524 total cases that occurred in the period 2003–2004 in the United States.

In considering age alone among the subjects, the researchers found that the greatest overall rate of bacteremic pneumonia was among adults ages 80 years and older, with a rate of 63.7 per 100,000. In considering race and ethnicity alone, the researchers found that the greatest overall percentage (24.2 per 100,000 people) of subjects with bacteremic pneumonia were Blacks of all ages, compared to the rate for Whites of all ages (10.1 per 100,000 people). This analysis did not include American Indians or Asians. Blacks ages 80 years and older had a very high rate of 79.4 cases of bacteremic pneumonia per 100,000.

Poverty levels were also considered and divided up into cases where less than 5% of the population were at the poverty level to the group in which 20% or more were at the poverty level. In general, the poorest group (or the group with 20% or more of its individuals living at the poverty level) had the highest rates of bacteremic pneumonia when considering rates for nearly every category.

LUNG ABSCESS

A lung abscess can be a complication of pneumonia. A lung abscess is a cavity in the lung that contains pus and is usually caused by bacteria such as *Staphylococcus aureus* or other gram-negative forms of bacteria. It is primarily a problem of adults and rarely is seen in children. The pathogens may be aspirated from the mouth during a period of unconsciousness. The usual symptoms are high fever, chest pain, cough, and unplanned weight loss.

Lung abscess is rarely caused by *Legionella pneumoniae*, but such cases have been identified by researchers. In an analysis by Chinese physicians that was published in the journal *Internal Medicine* in 2009, the researchers analyzed 62 cases of *Legionella*, including about half of the cases with hospital-acquired pneumonia and about half identified with community-acquired pneumonia. Nearly a third (27.4%) of the patients died.

The researchers noted that the most significant factor in the lung abscess patients was a prior treatment with cortiocosteroid drugs, and they speculated that the corticosteroid treatment received by about 70% of the study patients may have weakened their immune systems and made them susceptible to *Legionella*. The patients had been treated with corticosteroids because of an organ transplantation, blood cancer, an infection with the human immunodeficiency virus, or other disorders.[4]

A study of 252 patients diagnosed with a lung abscess over the period of 1968 to 2004, published in *Jornal Brasileiro de Pneumologia*, the official journal of the Brazilian Thoracic Society, by researchers José da Silva Moreira and colleagues, examined 209 male subjects and 43 female subjects; their average age was 41.4 years. Most of the subjects (70.2%) were alcoholics. The majority also had dental disease (82.5%). In addition, the majority (78.6%) of the subjects also had experienced a loss of consciousness on at least one occasion, particularly one that was caused by the abuse of alcohol. Most (65%) of the subjects were smokers. It is clear that these lifestyle choices (alcohol abuse and smoking) were likely key factors that contributed to the development of the lung abscess.[5]

ACUTE RESPIRATORY DISTRESS SYNDROME

First described in 1967 in the *Lancet*,[6] ARDS is a serious complication of pneumonia. It is also caused by trauma, pancreatitis, or aspiration pneumonia. According to the National Heart, Lung, and Blood Institute, ARDS is a lung condition that causes the oxygen levels in the blood to decrease. Other names for ARDS include noncardiac pulmonary edema, increased-permeability pulmonary edema, adult respiratory distress syndrome, and acute lung injury.

ARDS is dangerous to the body because organs such as the brain and the kidneys need oxygenated blood in order to function. Pneumonia is one cause of ARDS. Other causes are other infections and injuries. Most people who develop ARDS are already in the hospital. According to the National Institutes of Health, about a third of those with ARDS die. Of those who survive, many have problems with memory loss because of the lack of oxygen to the brain that they suffered when their lungs were not working well and when the brain was deprived of oxygen.[7]

Low blood oxygen levels, shortness of breath, rapid breathing, and a feeling that the individual cannot get enough air into the lungs are all symptoms of ARDS. ARDS is diagnosed with a chest X-ray, an arterial blood gas test (which shows the oxygen level of the blood), and sputum cultures (which culture the coughed up spit so that the source of the infection can be identified). In addition, other blood tests will be ordered as needed. A chest computerized tomography (CT) scan may also be ordered.

This complication of pneumonia (and some other disorders or conditions) is treated with oxygen therapy, medications such as antibiotics and painkillers, and extra fluids, usually administered intravenously, and is usually treated in the intensive care unit of the hospital. A ventilator will be used to help the person breathe until he or she can breathe unaided. If the ventilator is needed for more than a few days, a tracheostomy may be done, in which a cut is made in the neck to enable the physician to connect the breathing tube directly to the windpipe.

Individuals with ARDS are at risk for developing further complications such as a collapsed lung, scarring of the lungs, and blood clots.[8]

EMPYEMA

Empyema is a serious complication of pneumonia. It is characterized by a collection of pus outside the lung and within the chest cavity that contains the lungs, and it can include up to a pint or more of infected fluid, which places pressure upon the lungs.[9] Among children, empyema occurs most frequently in those younger than five years old.

Symptoms of empyema are chest pain (particularly when the person breathes in), sweating (especially at night), shortness of breath, chills, and fever. Diagnosis is made with a chest X-ray or a CT scan of the chest. A Gram's stain and culture of the fluid may also be done. A chest tube may be inserted through the chest wall to drain the pus.

In a Canadian study of 251 children with empyema that was associated with pneumonia, the average age of the children was six years. An identification of the microbe infecting the children was made in about a third of the cases and in only one case were there two pathogens: both *Streptococcus pneumoniae* and *Streptococcus pyogenes*. In the remaining children, one organism only was found: *S. pneumoniae* was the cause in 38 children; *S. pyogenes* in 20 children; *Staphylococcus aureus* in eight children; *S. milleri* in six; *Fusobacteria* in two children; and in one child each, the cause was *Mycobacterium tuberculosis*, *Eikenella corrodens*, and *Echinococcus*. The diagnosis of empyema was made within 24 hours of hospitalization in nearly two-thirds of the children, and it was made in 95% of the children by the fifth day of their hospital stay.

The researchers noted that most of the children were previously healthy. Most were treated with pain medication, as well as supplemental oxygen and a chest drain. The researchers further noted that the problem was disproportionately present in aboriginal (Native) children, who made up 18% of the patient population despite being less than about 3% of the Canadian population.[10]

DEATH: THE MOST SERIOUS COMPLICATION

Despite the ready access to antibiotics for most people in the United States, the CDC reports that about 55,000 people in the United States die each year from pneumonia and its complications.[11] Many people who died of pneumonia were hospitalized in an intensive care unit (ICU), and such individuals suffer up to a 50% death rate. Others die hospitalized in another part of the hospital, with up to an 8% death rate, according to Burke A. Cunha, M.D., author of *Pneumonia Essentials*.[12]

According to Paul Ellis Marik, in a chapter on CAP in the *Handbook of Evidence-Based Care*, the death rate of patients with CAP who are outpatients is 1 to 5%. But if patients with CAP are hospitalized, their death risk increases as high as 12%. If the patient becomes so sick that he or she needs care in an ICU, then the risk for death increases to 35%.[13]

In a study by Scott T. Micek and colleagues that compared the death rates of 639 hospitalized adults patients who were diagnosed with either CAP or health care–associated pneumonia (HCAP), the researchers found that about two-thirds of

ANEMIA WITH PNEUMONIA INCREASES DEATH RATE

Anemia can affect the outcome of patients who are hospitalized because of pneumonia. A study published in *BMC Pulmonary Medicine* of the daily hemoglobin levels among 1,893 hospitalized subjects found that one in three subjects who were hospitalized for CAP had at least mild anemia at admission while 3 out of 5 were anemic during their hospital stay. In addition, half of the subjects were discharged with a diagnosis of anemia. Anemia was most common among females, those with two or more illnesses, and those with poor outcomes of their illnesses. The researchers found that the combination of anemia and pneumonia increased the risk for death if hemogloblin levels were 10 grams per deciliter (g/dL) or less (moderate to severe anemia).[14]

HOSPITALIZATION FOR PNEUMONIA DECREASES LIFE SPAN FOR ALL AGES

Although it is known that elderly patients who are hospitalized for pneumonia have a higher risk of death, the effect of the hospitalization for pneumonia among adults younger than age 65 was unknown until researchers Laura M. Cecere and colleagues reported in 2010 in the publication *Respiration* on the outcome for 457 of 522 non-elderly subjects who were hospitalized for pneumonia. The researchers found that either admission to the hospital for HCAP or admission to the hospital for CAP increased the mortality risks among adults.

It was not that the hospitalization somehow caused their deaths but rather that these patients were sicker than individuals who were not hospitalized. In about half the cases, the human immunodeficiency virus (HIV) and cardiovascular disease were responsible for the deaths of the pneumonia patients, and in 12% of the cases chronic lung disease led to their deaths. In considering those subjects with CAP only, the leading cause of death was cardiovascular disease, accounting for 35%.[15]

the hospitalized patients had HCAP versus one-third who were hospitalized with CAP. They also found that the death rate was much higher for the HCAP patients; it was nearly 25% for the HCAP patients, compared with a death rate of about 9% for the CAP patients.[16] This is one form of verification of the worse prognosis of hospitalized HCAP patients versus CAP patients who need hospitalization.

It is also important to note that the pathogens causing pneumonia are often different for CAP patients than for HCAP patients. For example, according to Micek and colleagues, among the CAP patients who were admitted to the hospital, the most common pathogen was *Streptococcus pneumoniae*, a problem for nearly 41% of these CAP subjects. However, among the HCAP subjects, *Streptococcus pneumoniae* was a problem for only about 10% of these subjects. In addition, results from the Micek study showed that the largest single cause of pneumonia infection for the HCAP patients was methicillin-resistant *Staphylococcus aureus* (MRSA), accounting for about 31% of the HCAP subjects. (MRSA is a bacteria that is resistant to many antibiotics.) In contrast, the hospitalized CAP subjects had a much lower MRSA rate of 12%.

IDENTIFYING THE RIGHT ANTIBIOTIC THE FIRST TIME IS CRUCIAL TO PATIENTS WITH HCAP

It's always best to give an infected patient the right antibiotic the first time. But in the case of patients who develop pneumonia while they are in a hospital, or who reside at a nursing home and then are hospitalized with pneumonia, as well as patients receiving dialysis who develop pneumonia, giving them the right antibiotic the first time can mean the difference between life and death. In a study of 421 patients with HCAP, 396 patients survived beyond 48 hours, but the overall death rate of the survivors was still eventually a very high 21.5%. Analysis of the records revealed that those individuals who died were significantly more likely to have been treated with inappropriate antibiotics (37.6%) compared to the patients who survived and who were initially given inappropriate antibiotics (24.1%). The researchers noted that the wrong choice of the first antibiotic nearly tripled the risk for death.[17]

AFTEREFFECTS OF PNEUMONIA

Some individuals spring back to relatively normal functioning soon after their diagnosis, treatment, and recovery from pneumonia. Others, however, require further help to bring their level of functioning back to their former level. For example, an elderly person discharged from the hospital may need short-term nursing-home care and physical therapy for at least several weeks because the individual is still weak. Others may do well with home health care, in which nurses, physical therapists, and other assistants as needed can provide an evaluation of the individual's current health status, teach the individual specific exercises to build up the individual's physical strength, and offer other support identified by the physician or others.

6

Diagnosis, Treatment, and Prevention

Eva, 83, was coughing severely and painfully and she was also confused and upset, although her daughter told the hospital emergency room staff that Eva was normally lucid and competent. Her blood pressure was low and for some reason she was shaking although she had no fever. The emergency room staff ordered blood work and the phlebotomist struggled to hit a good vein to take enough blood. It was even harder to insert an intravenous tube. Eva kept saying she wanted to go home but it was clear to everyone but her that she needed to be admitted. Eva's daughter told her that everything would be all right.

Eva was admitted to the hospital with community-acquired pneumonia and she was treated with antibiotics intravenously as well as fluids to keep her hydrated and her blood pressure stable. Four days later she was much better and was released, but the doctor ordered home health services to visit the extremely fatigued Eva at home, and her daughter promised to check on her mother daily for the next two weeks. The doctor said that without the home health care and the frequent checks by her daughter, Eva would need to enter a nursing home for at least a two-week stay.

Doctors may suspect pneumonia based on the patient's symptoms, but they need to go through what is called a "differential diagnosis," a careful consideration of several possible diagnoses so that they can ask questions and order radiologic and laboratory tests, the physician can eliminate some possibilities and zero in on the true cause of the patient's suffering.

HOW PNEUMONIA IS DIAGNOSED

Pneumonia can often be strongly suspected by the patient's signs and symptoms, but a chest X-ray and basic laboratory tests are usually performed as well. The physical examination is another vital aspect of diagnosis. Diagnostic testing among patients with CAP depends on the patient and how ill he or she is. For example, all patients suspected of having pneumonia should receive a complete blood count, a chest X-ray, analysis of blood oxygen levels, and a complete metabolic profile. But patients who are severely ill—those who are immunocompromised or individuals who have serious anatomic problems with their lungs—should additionally receive a sputum culture, **blood cultures**, and other tests.

The Physical Examination

The doctor will review the patient's symptoms, check the patient's nose and throat, and listen to the patient's chest with a stethoscope to check for crackling sounds or any other unusual

WHEN OTHER DISEASES OR CONDITIONS MASQUERADE AS PNEUMONIA

When making a diagnosis, it is important for the physician to consider other illnesses or conditions that may appear to be pneumonia. For example, some drugs may cause symptoms that present as pneumonia, such as methotrexate or gold (used to treat rheumatoid arthritis), amiodarone (used to treat cardiac arrhythmias), or nitrofurantoin (an antibiotic). In addition, some diseases may present with symptoms similar to pneumonia, such as a pulmonary embolism (blood clot in the lungs), lung cancer, or tuberculosis.[1]

noises that can indicate that there is inflammation present in the lungs. The patient's past history is also reviewed; for example, the patient may have had a recent flu or other illness or could have recurrent bronchial or pneumonia issues, and if so, this could cause an elevated risk for the development of another infection. Patients may also have specific risk factors for the

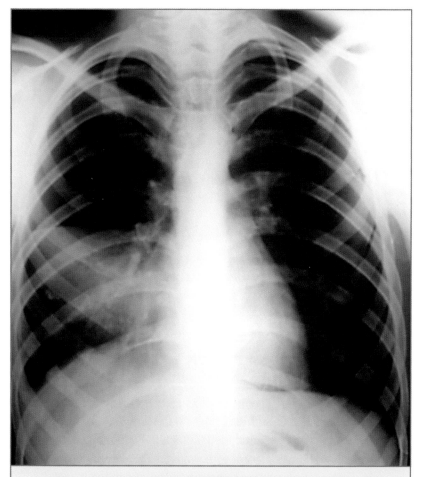

Figure 6.1 X-ray of chest of a patient showing bacterial pneumonia in the middle lobe of one lung (at center left, white area). (© Photo Researchers)

development of pneumonia, such as being a smoker and/or alcohol drinker as well as being of an advanced age.

The Chest X-Ray

A simple chest X-ray can detect most cases of pneumonia, although rarely, as with some atypical forms of pneumonia, the chest X-ray will be normal. Even with more common forms of pneumonia, when the X-ray is performed too early in the course of the disease, the findings may be negative despite the presence of pneumonia.

Laboratory Tests

Laboratory tests will also be run. For example, a complete blood count will provide data on red and white blood cell counts. An elevated white blood cell count often indicates the presence of a bacterial infection infection. The blood can also be cultured to determine whether the patient has bacteremia (bacteria within the bloodstream). Doctors can narrow down the type of pneumonia with further tests, such as an analysis of sputum. However, laboratory tests other than a complete blood count may be foregone if the doctor is convinced, based on the physical examination and the chest X-ray, that the patient has pneumonia.

A possible reason for the omission of the sputum test is that the doctor may assume that antibiotics that are prescribed immediately will probably clear up the infection before the test results come back. However, if the infection persists and the antibiotic does not appear to be working, a sputum analysis is probably in order. Also, if the infection is defined as a hospital-acquired pneumonia (HAP) or ventilator-associated pneumonia (VAP), then it is generally more likely that a less common pathogen has caused the pneumonia. A sputum analysis could help identify the pathogen that is causing the pneumonia, which will then help the doctor determine which antibiotic or other drug (such as an antiviral medication) should be prescribed. A **urinary antigen test** can also identify pneumonia.

Sputum Stain and Culture

A Gram's stain of the sputum can detect the presence of many bacteria that cause pneumonia. However, this test may not be useful if the patient has been on antibiotics beforehand. In addition, experts report that sputum can often be contaminated by saliva, and consequently a good enough quality of sputum is available in only about 40 to 60% of patients with CAP. If only patients with bacteremia and with purulent sputum are considered, then the quality of the sputum culture is more likely to be good.[2] Some studies have indicated that valid sputum samples were less common in elderly patients—43.1% versus 56.5% of valid samples in younger patients.[3] The reason for this may be that some older patients may have trouble complying with directions for the sputum test or they may have more difficulty spitting up the sample.

If it is taken prior to antibiotics however, and presuming the sample is a good one, the test has been found accurate in more than 80% of patients with pneumococcal pneumonia.[4] According to a joint statement issued by the Infectious Diseases Society of America and the American Thoracic Society, pretreatment sputum cultures should be obtained from those patients who have to be admitted to the intensive care unit of the hospital, as well as to other groups including those individuals with active alcohol abuse, those with severe lung disease, patients who have tested positive on the urinary antigen test for *Legionella*, and patients with pleural effusion (an accumulation of fluid between the lungs and the chest wall). In addition, patients who have failed antibiotic treatment should also have this test.[5]

The bronchoscopic evaluation yields a more accurate result, but it is an invasive test and is less likely to be performed on older patients, possibly because physicians are reluctant to perform the test on the elderly.

In his article on CAP, Steven Schmitt, M.D., notes that the sputum stain and culture are controversial tests but that they can be helpful to the physician when the patient has a compromised immune system or is extremely ill.[6]

Blood Culture

The blood may show the presence of bacteria (bacteremia) that can be identified in a culture, and thus the physician may order a blood culture. According to both the Infectious Diseases Society of America and the American Thoracic Society, pretreatment blood cultures should be ordered for those patients who are admitted to the intensive care unit of the hospital, those with leukopenia (an abnormally low level of white blood cells), those individuals who are active alcohol abusers, patients with chronic severe liver disease, patients with no spleen or whose spleen has failed, patients with pleural effusion, and patients with a positive pneumococcal urinary antigen test.[7]

Urinary Antigen Test

The urinary antigen test for adults can detect *Streptococcus pneumoniae* as well as *Legionella pneumophilia* and some other types of bacteria and fungi. Some forms of the test are

TESTS NEEDED BY PATIENTS WITH SEVERE COMMUNITY-ACQUIRED PNEUMONIA

Some tests may not be routinely ordered but are needed when patients are very ill with CAP, says Paul Ellis Marik in his 2010 book on critical care. According to Marik, patients with severe CAP need to receive a blood culture, urinary antigen tests for both *S. pneumoniae* and *Legionella pneumophila*, and a sputum culture. They should also be screened for the human immunodeficiency virus (HIV) and, if it is flu season, should receive a nasopharyngeal swab for flu.[8]

very rapid and can be run at the bedside of the patient within about 15 minutes. Another advantage is that it does not require experienced laboratory technicians to run the test.[9] The test for *S. pneumoniae* can detect all 23 of the primary different *S. pneumoniae* types that represent more than 90% of all infections with *Streptococcus pneumoniae*.

In an analysis of the urinary antigen test among 59 patients in 2006, the researchers found that the test was 89% positively predictive (which means that it accurately identified *S. pneumoniae* among those patients who actually were infected with this pathogen). The researchers also found that the urinary antigen test had a 93% negative predictive value—which means that in 93% of the cases where the test said that the person

USING A TEST TO DECIDE WHETHER TO HOSPITALIZE PNEUMONIA PATIENTS

When a doctor diagnoses CAP in an adult, he or she must then decide whether the person needs to be hospitalized. According to the Infectious Diseases Society of America and the American Thoracic Society in their consensus guidelines, the CURB-65 severity score is a good, simple test to help the doctor determine if hospital admission is best for a person with pneumonia. The elements of the test include "C" for confusion, "U" for a blood urea nitrogen of greater than 19 milligram per deciliter (mg/dL), "R" for a respiratory rate at or above 30 breaths per minute, and "B" for low blood pressure (a systolic blood pressure of less than 90 mm Hg or a diastolic blood pressure of equal to or less than 60 mm Hg or both). Last, the doctor considers whether the patient is age 65 or older.[10]

To ascertain the presence of confusion, an abbreviated mental status test is given and the patient is asked each of 10 questions. If they get each question right, then they did not have pneumonia, they really did not have it. These are considered very good results, and thus the test was recommended by researchers as a supplement to conventional laboratory tests for pneumonia.[11]

Pulse Oximetry and Arterial Blood Gases

Patients with pneumonia may develop very low blood oxygen levels (hypoxemia), and for this reason, when they are in the emergency room or hospitalized, their blood levels are monitored with **pulse oximetry** and/or laboratory tests for arterial blood gases. With pulse oximetry, a simple monitor, such as one that slips over the finger, measures blood oxygen levels. For greater accuracy, arterial blood can also be tested for oxygen

receive one point, for a possible maximum of 10 points. If the patient scores eight or less in the mental confusion tests, then they are regarded as confused. Questions include asking the patients their age, their date of birth, the current year, their address or current location, and so forth. The next step on the test is that if the patient is considered confused based on these criteria, then a score of one is given on the CURB-65.

One point is awarded for each of the CURB-65 criteria, for a maximum of five points. If the patient scores three to five, then he or she should be admitted to the hospital right away, possibly to intensive care. If the score is two, then a short inpatient hospital stay may be considered. If the patient scores a one or a zero, despite the presence of pneumonia, then the patient should be treated at home because this patient is considered at low risk for death.[12]

levels, which may be needed in the cases of severely ill patients. The arterial blood gas test can also determine if a patient who is receiving oxygen is reaching the correct blood oxygen level. Some pharmacies sell pulse oximetry meters so that individuals can check on their own blood oxygen levels.

Bronchoscopy

Using the fiber optics of the bronchoscope, physicians can visualize the affected area of the lung of the patient with pneumonia and can also take a sample from the bronchial area. The physician inserts the bronchoscope through the nose or mouth, then through the trachea and finally into the lungs. This test is more likely to be ordered if the patient has HAP or VAP. The doctor may also place saline solution in the bronchoscope to wash the lungs and enable the collection of samples of fluids and lung cells from the air sacs (alveoli) for further analysis. This washing part of the procedure is called a bronchoalveolar lavage. The bronchoscopy with broncho-alveolar lavage is more costly than laboratory tests or X-rays but is considered highly specific for determining the infect-ing pathogen.[11] This test also may be used if the patient is very ill and has not responded to medications prescribed for *S. pneumoniae*.

TREATMENT

Once pneumonia is diagnosed, it must be promptly treated with medications, rest, and other treatments, such as providing oxygen or inhaled corticosteroids. Hospitalization may also be needed. If the pathogen causing the pneumonia is a bacterium, then antibiotics are used to fight the disease. If the person has influenza, which may lead to pneumonia in high-risk groups, then antiviral drugs may be used.

Antiviral Medications

If it is a virus and in the very early stages of influenza infection, then **antivirals** may be administered. As of this writing in late

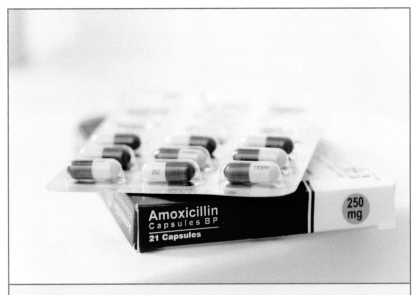

Figure 6.2 Bacterial pneumonia is treated with antibiotics such as amoxicillin. (© Photo Researchers)

2010, oseltamivir (Tamiflu) and zanamivir (Relenza) are the two antivirals that are recommended by the CDC for the treatment of sickness with influenza among those at risk for complications such as pneumonia.[14] Antivirals can help to shorten the course of a viral illness by a day or two and they can also help to prevent complications. It is generally best if the antiviral is started within the first 48 hours of the onset of symptoms; however, if the individual is at risk for complications, even taking an antiviral later than two days after symptoms have begun can be helpful. In general, oseltamivir and zanamivir are taken for five days.

Individuals who are most at risk for complications from the flu include the following groups: children younger than two, adults age 65 and older, women who are pregnant or who delivered their babies in the past two weeks, and individuals with asthma, heart failure, and chronic lung disease, as well as those with weak immune systems caused by diabetes or HIV.[15]

Antibiotic Drugs

There are numerous types of medications that may be effective against the pathogen causing pneumonia. If the causative organism is not known, a broad-spectrum antibiotic may be chosen, which would be effective against the frequently occurring *Streptococcus pneumoniae* as well as many other pathogens. According to physicians at the University of Maryland Medical Center Web site, the severity of the infection must be considered and whether the illness can be treated at home or whether the patient needs to be hospitalized. If the patient can be treated at home, oral antibiotics are given, while if the patient requires hospitalization, then intravenous antibiotics are usually administered.

The doctor should also consider whether the infection was community-acquired or hospital-acquired, which is another factor dictating the choice of antibiotics. Another factor is whether the patient with CAP has other serious

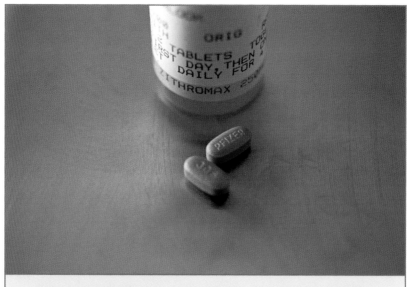

Figure 6.3 Azithromycin is one antibiotic alternative to penicillin. (© Photo Researchers)

diseases, such as diabetes, kidney disease, or heart disease and consequently should be given a fluoroquinolone drug, such as levofloxacin (Levaquin), gemifloxacin (Factive), or moxifloxacin (Avelox).[16]

There are many different types of antibiotics, and some are more effective than others at treating specific pathogens. For example, if the bacterium is believed to be *Streptococcus pneumoniae* and it is not a type of pathogen that has developed penicillin resistance (meaning the adaptive ability to survive treatment with penicillin), then it may be treated with penicillin G or amoxicillin. If the doctor does not wish to use these drugs, then alternative choices are drugs that are known as macrolides (such as azithromycin [Zithromax], clarithromycin [Biaxin], and erythromycin), cephalosporins (cefpodoxime [Vantin], cefprozil [Cefzil] or cefuroxime [Ceftin]), or other antibiotics.

However, if the *S. pneumoniae* is believed to be resistant to penicillin, which basically means that penicillin cannot kill the pathogen, then a drug in the fluoroquinolone class (levofloxacin, gemifloxacin, or moxifloxacin) may be chosen. Alternatively, penicillin-resistant *S. pneumoniae* may be treated with vancomycin, oral linezolid, or high doses of oral amoxicillin. In most cases, oral medication is given but sometimes parenteral (injected) drugs are administered to obtain faster action.

If the pathogen is known to be or believed to be *Legionella*, then drugs such as fluoroquinolone or azithromycin (Zithromax) may be chosen. In some cases, a tetracycline drug such as doxycycline is the preferred antibiotic. See Table 6.1 for a listing of different types of pneumonia-causing organisms and the preferred antimicrobial as well as alternatives that may be given.

Rest

Most patients with pneumonia are fatigued and will agree to stay in bed; however, some try to continue working or caring

Table 6.1   Recommended Antimicrobial Therapy for Specific Pathogens

Organism	Preferred Antimicrobial(s)	Alternative Antimicrobial(s)
Streptococcus pneumoniae		
Penicillin nonresistant	Penicillin G, amoxicillin	Macrolide, cephalosporins (oral [cefpodoxime, cefprozil, cefuroxime, cefdinir, cefditoren] or parenteral [cefuroxime, ceftriaxone, cefotaxime]), clinidamycin, doxycycline, respiratory fluoroquinolone
Penicillin resistant	Agents chosen on the basis of susceptibility, including cefotaxime, ceftriaxone, fluoroquinolone	Vancomycin, linezolid, high-dose amoxicillin
Haemophilus influenzae		
Non-ß-lactamase producing	Amoxicillin	Fluoroquinolone, doxycycline, azithromycin, clarithromycin
ß-Lactamase producing	Second- or third-generation cephalosporoin, amoxicillin-clavulanate	Fluoroquinolone, doxycycline, azithromycin, clarithromycin
Mycoplasma pneumoniae/ Chlamydophila pneumoniae	Macrolide, a tetracycline	A fluoroquinolone
Legionella species	Fluoroquinolone, azithromycin	Doxycycline
Chlamydophila psittaci	A tetracycline	A macrolide
Coxiella burnetii	A tetracycline	A macrolide
Francisella tularensis	Doxycycline	Gentamicin, streptomycin
Yersinisa pestis	Streptomycin, gentamicin	Doxycycline, fluoroquinolone
Bacillus anthracis (inhalation)	Ciprofloxacin, levofloxacin, doxycycline (usually with second agent)	Other fluoroquinolones; ß-lactam, if susceptible; rifampin; clindamycin; chloramphenicol
Enterobacteriaceae	Third-generation cephalosporin, carbapenem (drug of choice if extended-specific ß-lactamase producer)	ß-Lactam/ ß-lactamase inhibitor, fluoroquinolone

Table 6.1 (*continued*)

Organism	Preferred Antimicrobial(s)	Alternative Antimicrobial(s)
Pseudomonas aeruginosa	Antipseudomonal ß-lactam **plus** (ciprofloxacin or levofloxacin or aminoglycoside)	Aminoglycoside **plus** (ciprofloxacin or levofloxacin), antipseudomal carbapenem
Burkholderia pseudomallei	Carbapenem, ceftadime	Fluoroquinolone, trimethoprim/sulfamethoxazole (TMP-SMX)
Acinetobacter species	Carbapenem	Cephalosporin-aminoglycoside, ampicillin-sulbactam, colistin
Staphylococcus aureus		
Methicillin susceptible	Antistaphylococcal penicillin	Cefazolin, clindamycin, ceftriaxone
Methicillin resistant	Vancomycin or linezolid	Trimethoprim/sulfamethoxazole (TMP-SMX)
Bordetella pertussis	Macrolide	Trimethoprim/sulfamethoxazole (TMP-SMX)
Anaerobe (aspiration)	ß-Lactam/ ß-lactamase inhibitor, clindamycin	Carbapenem
Influenza virus	Oseltamivir or zanamivir	
Mycobacterium tuberculosis	Isoniazid plus rifampin plus ethambutol plus pyrazinamide	
Coccidioides species	For uncomplicated infection in a normal host, no therapy generally recommended; for therapy, itraconazole, fluconazole	Amphotericin B
Histoplasmosis	Itraconazole	Amphotericin B
Blastomycosis	Itraconazole	Amphotericin B

for their children. Unfortunately, if the individual is not treated with medication, then he or she is likely to spread the pathogens that caused the pneumonia to others at work and at home. Bed rest is an important element of recovery from pneumonia.

Oxygen Therapy

Pneumonia patients who have difficulty breathing may need oxygen therapy, which is usually administered in the hospital with the use of nasal cannulae, or small tubes that are inserted into the nostrils and which are connected to an oxygen outlet. Oxygen levels are frequently measured among hospitalized patients with pneumonia. Oxygen therapy has been used with pneumonia patients for about a hundred years.

Nebulization Treatments

Liquid medications, including some antibiotics, that are aerosolized with the use of a nebulizing compressor may be administered to patients with pneumonia to help clear the lungs and also to make breathing easier, because these inhaled corticosteroids decrease airway inflammation and make it easier for the patient to breathe. These treatments may be needed at multiple intervals during a hospital stay by a patient with pneumonia, and they may also need to be continued at home as well, depending on the recommendations of the physician.

Hospitalization

Elderly individuals, infants and toddlers, and the immunocompromised are the most likely to need hospitalization to prevent complications that can develop from pneumonia. Hospitalization may be required to keep the patient alive by providing the intensive care, medical expertise, and technological access that families are unable to provide. For example, nurses in the hospital can monitor the patient on a 24-7 basis, and if the patient's vital signs fall dangerously low, nurses can identify and treat the problem and obtain the physician's advice rapidly.

PREVENTING PNEUMONIA

Pneumococcal pneumonia is often preventable, particularly among the elderly, yet less than two-thirds of all adults in the United States ages 65 and older are immunized against pneumonia, and the figures are even lower for Hispanic and African-American adults. Most immunized adults ages 65 and older are white (65% of this population), while only 44.5% of

WASHING HANDS, EVEN IN AN EMERGENCY SITUATION

Hand washing can remove many transmissible pathogens that can cause pneumonia as well as other microbes that are picked up in the course of a busy person's daily life, whether at home, work, or in the many stops along the way that may occur. As a rule, the hands should be washed after each time a person uses the toilet, but more frequent hand washing is also recommended.

Washing one's hands is much more difficult when an individual is in an emergency situation, such as after a hurricane or other disaster, when the power is often out and water may be at a premium or not available at all. In such cases, the CDC still advises washing the hands with soap and warm water for 20 seconds and using alcohol-based products such as hand sanitizers or alcohol wipes when soap and water is not available. Even during a disaster, the CDC says that hands should be washed before preparing or eating food, after changing diapers or cleaning a child who has toileted, before and after caring for an ill person, after blowing the nose, coughing or sneezing, after handling an animal or animal waste, after handling garbage, both before and after treating a cut or wound, after handing items contaminated by flood water or sewage, and after handling uncooked foods, especially raw meat, poultry, or fish.

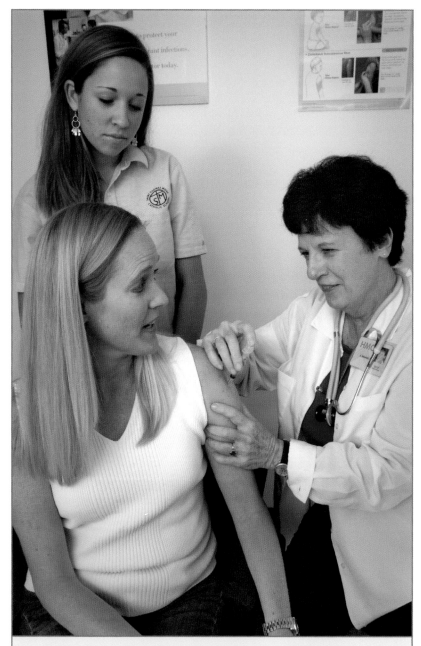

Figure 6.4 **Flu vaccination is one key method of preventing pneumonia. (Centers for Disease Control and Prevention)**

elderly African Americans and 40% of elderly Hispanics are immunized against pneumonia. As a result, these unimmunized groups have an elevated risk for developing pneumonia.

The Flu Vaccination

Getting an influenza shot is an important preventive measure against the contracting of pneumonia, because flu can often develop into pneumonia among vulnerable populations. According to the CDC, some groups of individuals who do not get the flu shot are at high risk for developing complications from flu, such as pneumonia, ear infections, and bronchitis.[17] Such groups include children under age five, but particularly children two years old and younger, as well as adults ages 65 and older, and pregnant women. A nasal form of the immunization can be used for healthy people, age 2 to 49.

Individuals with some diseases have a high risk for developing complications from the flu if they do not get vaccinated, such as those with asthma, diabetes, chronic lung disease, chronic obstructive pulmonary disease (COPD), and cystic fibrosis.

In addition, people who have been diagnosed with heart disease (such as congestive heart failure, congenital heart disease, and coronary artery disease) have a high risk for becoming very

CHILDREN UNDER AGE FIVE DIRECTLY BENEFIT FROM VACCINATION FOR PNEUMOCOCCAL DISEASE

According to the CDC, before children were vaccinated for pneumonia, the rate of invasive pneumococcal disease (IPD) for children under five in the United States was 98.7 per 100,000 in 1999. In 2005, that rate had dropped substantially to 3.4 per 100,000.[18] Invasive pneumococcal disease includes pneumonia, bacteremia, or meningitis that is caused by *Streptococcus pneumoniae*.

ill from the flu and for developing complications, a risk that is also shared by individuals with diabetes, kidney disorders, liver disorders, metabolic disorders, those individuals who are morbidly obese (with a body mass index of 40 or greater and who are about 100 pounds overweight or greater), and those individuals ages 19 years and younger who are receiving long-term aspirin therapy.[19]

Each year, a new flu shot is needed because the influenza virus changes constantly, and consequently, the general population needs to "keep up" by receiving the latest vaccine. However, many people fail to obtain an annual flu vaccination, including some people at high risk for complications from flu. According to the CDC, however, the group that had the highest rate of receiving a flu shot in 2008 was those individuals who were ages 65 and older, who had an immunization rate of 67%. This is up from 66.4% in 2007. Individuals ages 18 to 49 had the lowest overall immunization rate, at 20%. Individuals who were ages 50 to 64 had a 39.5% rate of an annual flu injection.[20] See Table 6.2 for further information.

The Pneumococcal Injection

The pneumococcal injection, also known as the pneumonia shot, is effective against several serotypes of S. pneumoniae. It protects people 65 and older as well as those with such health problems as alcoholism, HIV/AIDS, diabetes, and sickle-cell disease, according to the CDC. In addition, individuals with health issues involving their lungs, heart, liver, or kidneys should also obtain a pneumococcal shot. Most people need only one shot in their lifetime, but sometimes a booster of the pneumonia vaccine is needed after five years from the last shot. The flu shot will protect against influenza but will not protect individuals against the multiple other pathogens that can develop into pneumonia. That is why the pneumonia shot is needed.

People who receive the pneumonia shot have a lower risk of getting pneumococcal pneumonia, and the only side effect that may occur may be some minor redness or swelling at the injection site, which is gone within a few days.

Table 6.2 Self-Reported Influenza Vaccination Coverage Trends Among Adults by Age Group, Risk Group, Race/Ethnicity, Health-Care Worker Status, and Pregnancy Status by Percent, 2001–2008: United States, National Health Interview Survey (NHIS)

Characteristics	2001	2002	2003	2004	2005	2006	2007	2008
Age Group								
18–49	15.1	16.3	16.8	17.9	10.4	15.5	17.7	20.0
50–64	32.1	34.0	36.8	35.9	22.9	33.1	36.2	39.5
≥65	63.0	65.6	65.5	64.6	59.6	64.1	66.4	67.0
Age by Risk Status								
18–49								
High Risk	20.9	23.1	24.2	26.0	18.1	24.5	27.2	29.8
Not High Risk	14.0	15.3	15.8	16.6	9.1	14.1	16.3	18.4
50–64								
High Risk	40.9	43.6	46.3	45.5	33.9	44.4	46.0	49.6
Not High Risk	28.2	29.8	32.7	32.1	17.8	28.2	32.3	35.2
Age by Race/Ethnicity								
18–49								
White Not Hispanic	15.5	16.9	18.0	19.8	11.1	16.6	19.0	21.6
Black Not Hispanic	15.0	15.7	16.9	14.3	9.8	14.8	14.6	17.4
Hispanic	11.9	12.4	11.8	11.6	7.8	11.0	13.9	14.9
Asian/Pacific Islander Hispanic	17.4	19.7	18.1	21.5	9.0	20.2	20.5	23.8
50–64								
White Not Hispanic	34.6	35.8	38.8	38.3	24.5	34.8	38.2	41.5
Black Not Hispanic	23.2	28.0	28.4	26.0	19.9	28.2	29.1	35.8
Hispanic	22.1	25.7	27.3	27.7	15.4	25.0	27.0	29.4
Asian/Pacific Islander	20.6	31.0	31.7	33.7	12.7	27.7	31.4	33.0
65 and older								
White Not Hispanic	65.4	68.6	68.7	67.3	63.2	67.2	69.0	69.8
Black Not Hispanic	48.1	49.6	48.0	45.4	39.7	46.5	55.4	50.6

Table 6.2 (*continued*)

Characteristics	2001	2002	2003	2004	2005	2006	2007	2008
Hispanic	51.9	48.5	45.4	54.6	41.7	44.8	52.1	54.5
Asian/Pacific Islander	57.5	57.8	63.6	52.7	56.1	61.4	62.7	58.8
Age by Diabetes Status								
18–49								
With Diabetes	28.6	31.9	36.4	34.0	29.5	35.0	30.0	37.0
Without Diabetes	14.7	15.9	16.4	17.4	9.8	14.9	17.4	19.5
50–64								
With Diabetes	47.7	46.8	51.6	48.9	40.3	51.0	45.4	53.7
Without Diabetes	30.1	32.4	35.0	34.3	20.5	30.6	34.9	37.3
Age by Asthma Status								
18–49								
With Asthma	26.6	23.9	28.9	28.4	21.5	24.6	30.4	30.7
Without Asthma	14.6	14.6	16.4	17.5	9.9	15.2	17.2	19.6
50–64								
With Asthma	41.9	51.0	47.9	52.4	40.2	46.8	57.9	50.8
Without Asthma	31.8	31.8	36.3	35.3	22.2	32.5	35.4	39.1

Source: Adapted from Centers for Disease Control and Prevention. "Self-reported Influenza Vaccination Coverage Trends 1989–2008 Among Adults by Age Group, Risk Group, Race/Ethnicity, Health-Care Worker Status, and Pregnancy Status, United States, National Health Interview Survey (NHIS). Available online at http://www.cdc.gov/flu/professionals/vaccination/pdf/NHIS89_08fluvaxtrendtab.pdf. Accessed November 19, 2010.

Table 6.2 shows the characteristics of people who obtain the pneumonia vaccine. For example, among the age characteristic, there is a high of 60.1% among those ages 65 and older. Table 6.4 shows common reasons given to avoid receiving the flu or pneumonia vaccine, and the actual realities of the situation. For example, people may say they have not had the flu for years. However, the reality is that this may be the year that they actually do contract the flu unless they are immunized.

Table 6.3   Self-Reported Pneumococcal Vaccination Coverage Trends Among Adults by Age Group, Risk Group, Race/Ethnicity/Health-Care Worker Status, and Pregnancy Status by Percent, 2001–2008: United States, National Health Interview Survey (NHIS)

Characteristics	2001	2002	2003	2004	2005	2006	2007	2008
Age Group								
18–49	6.0	5.6	5.6	5.7	5.8	5.7	5.3	6.8
50–64	15.3	16.3	16.7	17.2	17.1	18.2	17.3	18.5
≥65	53.8	55.7	55.6	56.8	56.2	57.1	57.7	60.1
Age by Risk Status								
18–49								
High Risk	10.3	10.7	12.6	12.6	15.0	13.5	16.0	16.0
Not High Risk	5.3	5.0	4.7	4.8	4.5	4.7	4.1	5.5
50–64								
High Risk	26.7	28.8	29.2	30.2	30.6	32.5	32.2	33.9
Not High Risk	10.5	11.1	11.7	11.9	11.1	12.0	11.3	12.0
Age by Race/Ethnicity								
18–49								
White Not Hispanic	5.9	5.7	5.5	6.1	6.1	6.0	5.7	7.3
Black Not Hispanic	8.1	6.3	7.9	7.0	6.9	6.7	5.3	7.0
Hispanic	4.4	4.3	4.1	3.1	3.9	3.9	3.8	4.8
Asian/Pacific Islander	5.5	5.4	5.7	4.7	3.3	5.9	6.8	5.0
50–64								
White Not Hispanic	16.6	17.6	17.9	18.5	18.5	19.4	18.1	19.3
Black Not Hispanic	12.6	14.0	14.6	14.6	15.9	18.6	17.7	21.1
Hispanic	7.9	8.9	10.0	10.6	8.9	11.3	12.8	11.6
Asian/Pacific Islander	N/A	9.4	n/a	11.5	12.2	N/A	N/A	N/A
≥65								
White Not Hispanic	57.8	60.3	59.6	60.9	60.7	62.0	62.2	64.3
Black Not Hispanic	34.3	37.2	36.7	38.5	40.5	35.5	44.1	44.6

Table 6.3 (*continued*)

Characteristics	2001	2002	2003	2004	2005	2006	2007	2008
Hispanic	32.9	27.1	31.0	33.7	27.5	33.4	31.8	36.4
Asian/Pacific Islander	27.6	32.2	36.2	31.1	31.0	26.5	41.4	43.2
18–49 High Risk by Race/Ethnicity								
White Not Hispanic	10.4	10.9	13.1	13.4	16.0	14.2	17.5	17.2
Black Not Hispanic	10.3	10.3	15.9	13.0	15.3	12.1	13.3	11.5
Hispanic	10.0	10.1	7.4	6.6	9.2	8.5	12.5	12.9
50–64 High Risk by Race/Ethnicity								
White Not Hispanic	28.9	31.4	31.0	31.9	32.8	35.2	33.3	35.8
Black Not Hispanic	22.8	23.4	26.8	27.0	26.9	33.3	31.0	33.7
Hispanic	11.4	18.1	17.9	21.9	19.3	16.6	24.8	19.6
Age by Diabetes Status								
18–49								
With Diabetes	14.7	13.9	17.8	17.5	22.9	17.3	21.5	24.5
Without Diabetes	5.7	5.4	5.3	5.4	5.2	5.4	4.9	6.2
50–64								
With Diabetes	33.5	31.9	37.2	36.8	36.9	41.1	34.3	36.4
Without Diabetes	13.1	14.4	14.2	14.7	14.4	15.0	15.0	15.7

Source: Adapted from the Centers for Disease Control and Prevention. "Self-reported Pneumococcal Vaccination Coverage Trends 1989–2008 Among Adults by Age Group, Risk Group, Race/Ethnicity, Health-Care Worker Status, and Pregnancy Status, United States, National Health Interview Survey (NHIS)." Available online at www.cdc.gov/flu/professionals/pdf/NHIS89_08ppvvaxtrendtab.pdf. Accessed January 9, 2011.

LIFESTYLE CHANGES

Most individuals can decrease their risk for contracting pneumonia by making lifestyle changes such as ending a smoking habit, drinking less alcohol, exercising more, and improving their daily diet.

Table 6.4   Reasons Why People Don't Get Flu or Pneumonia Shots vs. Realities

Reasons for Not Getting Flu/Pneumonia Shots	Realities
I haven't had the flu in years.	You still could get the flu this year.
I'll get the flu if I get a shot.	The flu shot cannot cause the flu.
I don't have the time.	Do you have the time to be sick for three or four days with the flu?
I don't have the money.	Flu shots are inexpensive and sometimes are free, as for Medicare recipients.
I got a flu shot last year.	Flu shots must be received each year to be effective.

Stop Smoking

An excellent preventive action to the development of pneumonia—as well as a host of other illnesses up to and including lung cancer—is for people who smoke to stop smoking as soon as possible. With cessation of smoking, the lungs begin to recover from all the particles left behind by smoking. Some people find quitting smoking relatively easy, but most find it difficult. However, with the aid of nicotine replacement aids, and medication specifically designed to decrease the urge to smoke such as Zyban (bupropion), most people can successfully kick the habit.

Cut Back on Alcohol Consumption

Although moderate drinking, such as having a single glass of wine with dinner, may improve health, excessive alcohol consumption is very harmful. It leads to vitamin and mineral deficiencies, including deficiencies in vitamin A, vitamin C, and vitamin B1 [thiamine] as well as deficiencies of magnesium, and zinc. Alcoholism may also cause multiple health problems such as anemia, some forms of cancer (such as esophageal cancer, oral cancer, and cancer of the larynx), and cardiovascular disease such as heart attack and stroke. Individuals who are alcoholics also have an increased risk for infections, and some

PNEUMONIA VACCINE SHOULD BE GIVEN AT LEAST TWO WEEKS BEFORE SOME PROCEDURES

According to the CDC, the pneumococcal vaccination should be given at least two weeks before some procedures are performed, such as a splenectomy (the removal of the spleen) or a cochlear implant (an implant that is given to deaf people to enable them to hear). In addition, pneumococcal vaccination should be given at least two weeks before the start of chemotherapy for cancer or other immunosuppressive therapies, whenever possible.[21]

research indicates that nearly half of patients admitted to hospitals for pneumonia are alcoholics.[22]

Consider Changes in Nutrition or Diet That May Help

Sometimes a dietary change can be helpful in decreasing the risk for contracting pneumonia, such as adopting a diet that is high in fiber, and that is also replete with vegetables and fruit. Individuals should also drink plenty of water to help flush out germs that can otherwise proliferate and lead to infections.

SUMMARY AND FUTURE OUTLOOK

Pneumonia is clearly a major problem for many people today, especially with the aging population in the United States. However, the use of preventive measures, such as immunizations against flu and pneumonia, can help to reduce the numbers of afflicted people. In addition, preventive measures, such as giving up smoking and only drinking alcohol in moderation (or not at all), will decrease the incidence of pneumonia in the general adult population of the United States.

Another serious and emerging problem is that increasing numbers of pathogens have developed a resistance to existing antibiotics, and doctors and researchers fear the development of super-infections that are even more resistant to the antibiotic arsenal currently available. Researchers actively seek new antibiotics for the future threats that loom on the horizon. According to a 2010 statement from the Infectious Diseases Society of America (which included a discussion of all infections and not just pneumonia):

> Antibiotic resistance is a serious public health, patient care and safety, and national security issue. Antibiotic-resistant infections are extremely difficult to treat and frequently recur. These infections result in tremendous pain, suffering, and disfigurement in adults, children and infants, and have caused millions of deaths worldwide. Hospital-acquired antibiotic-resistant infections currently kill nearly one hundred thousand Americans each year (this does not include infections acquired outside of hospitals) and have been estimated to cost the U.S. health care system between $21 billion and $34 billion annually.[23]

It is also hoped that children in less-developed countries will be vaccinated against pneumonia, a scourge of countries in Africa and Asia. There are indicators of good progress; for example, in 2009, a national program of childhood vaccination was launched in Gambia, and the minister of health, Dr. Mariatou Jallow, gave the first dosage of the vaccine to a child in a rural clinic. The World Health Organization reported that severe pneumonia causes one of six deaths of children in Gambia. Vaccination of children should help dramatically decrease that rate.[24]

Notes

Chapter 1

1. Burke A. Cunha, *Pneumonia Essentials*, 3d ed. (Boston: Jones and Bartlett Publishers, 2010).
2. Centers for Disease Control and Prevention, "Pneumococcal Disease," www.cdc.gov/vaccines/pubs/pinkbook/downloads/pneumo.pdf (accessed November 12, 2010).
3. Cunha, *Pneumonia Essentials*.
4. Justin L. Ranes, Steven Gordon, and Alejandro C. Arroliga, "Hospital-Acquired, Health Care-Associated, and Ventilator-Associated Pneumonia," Cleveland Clinic Disease Management Project, www.clevelandclinicmeded.com/medicalpubs/diseasemanagement/infectious-disease/health-care-associated-pneumonia (accessed November 20, 2010).
5. Brad Spellberg, "Testimony of the Infectious Diseases Society of America (IDSA): Antibiotic Resistance: Promoting Critically Needed Antibiotic Research and Development and Appropriate Use ('Stewardship') of These Precious Drugs," Given Before the House Committee on Energy and Commerce Subcommittee on Health, June 9, 2010, www.idsociety.org/WorkArea/DownloadAsset.aspx?id=16656 (accessed January 10, 2011).
6. Cunha, *Pneumonia Essentials*.
7. Lionel A. Mandell, et al., "Infectious Diseases Society of American/American Thoracic Society Consensus Guidelines on the Management of Community-Acquired Pneumonia in Adults," *Clinical Infectious Diseases* 44 (2007): S27–S72.
8. Frederic Silverblatt, "Managing Health Care Facility Associated Pneumonias: Diagnosis, Treatment and Prevention," *Medicine & Health Rhode Island* 93, no. 7 (2010): 201–203.
9. MedlinePlus. "Hospital-Acquired Pneumonia," www.nlm.nih.gov/medlineplus/ency/article/000146.htm (accessed November 20, 2010).
10. National Institutes of Health, MedlinePlus, "Hospital-Acquired Pneumonia," www.nlm.nih.gov/medlineplus/ency/article/000146.htm (accessed September 23, 2010).
11. Antoni Torres, Miguel Ferrer, and Joan Ramón Badia, "Treatment Guidelines and Outcomes of Hospital-Acquired and Ventilator-Associated Pneumonia," *Clinical Infectious Diseases* 51, supplement 1 (2010): S48–S54.
12. Alvaro Rea-Neto, et al., "Diagnosis of Ventilator-Associated Pneumonia: A Systematic Review of the Literature," *Critical Care* 12 (2008), ccforum.com/content/12/2/R56 (accessed October 29, 2010).
13. Tamara Pilishvili, et al., "Chapter 11: Pneumococcal Disease," in *VPD Surveillance Manual*, 4th ed. (Atlanta: Centers for Disease Control and Prevention, 2008), www.cdc.gov/vaccines/pubs/surv-manual/chpt11-pneumo.pdf (accessed September 22, 2010).
14. Mandell, et al., "Consensus Guidelines."
15. Yana Vinogradova, Julia Hippisley-Cox, and Carol Coupland, "Identification of New Risk Factors for Pneumonia: Population-Based Case Control Study," *British Journal of General Practice* 567 (October 2009): 716–717.
16. Brendon R. Nolt, et al., "Vital-Sign Abnormalities as Predictors of Pneumonia in Adults with Acute Cough Illness," *American Journal of Emergency Medicine* 25, no. 6 (2007): 631–636.

Chapter 2

1. Centers for Disease Control and Prevention, "Pneumococcal Disease."
2. Solomon Solis, Cohen, "Recent Improvements in the Quinin Treatment of Lobar and Lobular Pneumonia," *Journal of the American Medical Association* 61, no. 2 (1913): 107–110.
3. Edward S. Mills, *The Diagnosis and Treatment of Pneumonia* (New York: Oxford University Press, 1939).
4. S. L. Abbot, "The Stimulating Treatment of Pneumonia," *Boston Medical and Surgical Journal* 136, no. 2 (1897): 37–38.
5. Mark S. Gold, and Christine Adamec, *The Encyclopedia of Alcoholism and*

Alcohol Abuse (New York: Facts On File, 2010).

6. Leath Lawrence, "Bloodletting: An Early Treatment Used by Barbers, Surgeons," *Cardiology Today*, September 1, 2008, www.cardiologytoday.com/view.aspx?rid=31588 (accessed November 20, 2010).

7. Gilbert R. Seigworth, "A Brief History of Bloodletting: Bloodletting Over the Centuries," *New York State Journal of Medicine* (1980): 2,022–2,028, www.pbs.org/wnet/redgold/printable/p_bloodlettinghistory.html (accessed September 27, 2010).

8. George E. Rennie, "Clinical Remarks on the Open-Air Treatment of Acute Pneumonia," *British Medical Journal* (1907): 495–496.

9. Rennie, "Open-Air Treatment of Acute Pneumonia."

10. Everett A. Bates, "Thoughts on the Treatment of Pneumonia," *Boston Medical and Surgical Journal* (1917): 293–296.

11. Lewis D. Hoppe, and William T. Freeman, "The Treatment of Pneumonia in Children with Mercurochrome Intravenously," *Southern Medical Journal* 17, no. 11 (1925): 784–787.

12. Powel Kazanjian, "Changing Interest among Physicians toward Pneumococcal Vaccination throughout the Twentieth Century," *Journal of the History of Medicine and Allied Sciences* 59, no. 4 (2004): 555–587.

13. Ibid.

14. J. Murray Kinsman, et al., "The Treatment of Pneumonia with Sulfonamides and Penicillin," *Journal of the American Medical Association* 128, no. 17 (1945): 1219–1224.

15. Kazanjian, "Changing Interest among Physicians toward Pneumococcal Vaccination throughout the Twentieth Century."

16. Ibid.

17. Immunization Action Coalition, "Pneumococcal Vaccine: Questions & Answers," www.vaccineinformation.org/pneumochild/qandavax.asp (accessed September 24, 2010).

18. F. T. Cutts, et al., "Efficacy of Nine-Valent Pneumococcal Conjugate Vaccine Against Pneumonia and Invasive Pneumococcal Disease in The Gambia: Randomised, Double-Blind, Placebo-Controlled Trial," *Lancet* 365, no. 9,465 (2005): 1,139–1,146.

19. National Institute of Allergy and Infectious Diseases, "The Gambia Pneumococcal Vaccine Trial," April 7, 2010, www.niaid.nih.gov/topics/bacterialinfections/clinical/gambia/Pages/GambiaPneumococcalVaccineTrial.aspx (accessed November 8, 2010); Cutts, "Nine-Valent Pneumococcal Conjugate Vaccine."

20. Centers for Disease Control and Prevention, "Pneumococcal Disease," www.cdc.gov/vaccines/pubs/pinkbook/downloads/pneumo.pdf (accessed September 27, 2010).

21. Immunization Action Coalition, "Pneumococcal Vaccine."

22. Immunization Action Coalition, "Pneumococcal Vaccine."

Chapter 3

1. National Institute of Allergy and Infectious Diseases, *Understanding Microbes in Sickness and in Health*, September 2009, www.niaid.nih.gov/topics/microbes/documents/microbesbook.pdf (accessed September 20, 2010).

2. Thomas M. File, Jr., "The Science of Selecting Antimicrobials for Community-Acquired Pneumonia (CAP)," *Journal of Managed Care Pharmacy* 15, no. 2, supplement (2009): S5–S11.

3. Walter Hampl and Thomas Mertens, "Viral Pathogens and Epidemiology, Detection, Therapy and Resistance," in Norbert Suttorp, et al., eds. *Community-Acquired Pneumonia* (Basel, Germany: Birkhäuser Verlag, 2007), 27–56.

4. National Heart, Lung, and Blood Institute, "What Causes Pneumonia," www.nhlbi.nih.gov/health/cdi/Diseases/pnu/pnu_causes.html (accessed October 22, 2010).

5. Penelope H. Denney, "Community-Acquired Pneumonia in Children,"

Medicine & Health Rhode Island 93, no. 7 (2010): 211–215.

6. Centers for Disease Control and Prevention, "Streptococcus pneumoniae," www.cdc.gov/ncidod/aip/research/spn.html (accessed October 23, 2010).

7. Reinhard Marre, "Detection of Respiratory Bacterial Pathogens," in Norbert Suttorp, et al., eds., *Community-Acquired Pneumonia* (Basel, Germany: Birkhäuser Verlag, 2007), 15–25.

8. Ken B. Waites, et al., "Pathogenesis of Mycoplasma Pneumoniae Infections: Adaptive Immunity, Innate Immunity, Cell Biology, and Virulence Factors," in Norbert Suttorp, et al., eds. *Community-Acquired Pneumonia* (Basel, Germany: Birkhäuser Verlag, 2007), 183–199.

9. Centers for Disease Control and Prevention, "Mycoplasma Pneumoniae," http://www.cdc.gov/ncidod/dbmd/diseaseinfo/mycoplasmapneum_t.htm (accessed January 19, 2010).

10. Waites, "Pathogenesis of Mycoplasma Pneumoniae Infections."

11. Leon G. Smith, "Mycoplasma Pneumonia and Its Complications," *Infectious Disease Clinics of North America* 34 (201): 57–60.

12. Ibid.

13. Matthias Krüll and Norbert Suttorp, "Pathogenesis of Chlamydophila Pneumoniae Infections—Epidemiology, Immunity, Cell Biology, Virulence Factors," in Norbert Suttorp, et al., eds. *Community-Acquired Pneumonia* (Basel, Germany: Birkhäuser Verlag, 2007), 83–110.

14. Almudena Burillo and Emilio Bouza, "Chlamydophila Pneumoniae," *Infectious Disease Clinics of North America* 24, no. 1 (2010): 61–71.

15. John E. Stupka, "Community-Acquired Pneumonia in Elderly Patients," *Aging Health* 5, no. 5 (2009): 763–774.

16. Krüll and Suttorp, "Pathogenesis of Chlamydophila Pneumoniae Infections."

17. Ibid.

18. Dina M. Bitar, et al., "Legionnaires' Disease and Its Agent *Legionella Pneu-*

mophila," in Norbert Suttorp, et al., eds. *Community-Acquired Pneumonia* (Basel, Germany: Birkhäuser Verlag, 2007), 111–138.

19. Ibid.

20. Marre, "Detection of Respiratory Bacterial Pathogens."

21. Stupka, "Community-Acquired Pneumonia in Elderly Patients."

22. Tara N. Palmore, et al., "A Cluster of Nosocomial Legionnaire's Disease Linked to a Contaminated Hospital Decorative Water Fountain," *Infection Control and Hospital Epidemiology* 30, no. 8 (2009): 764–768.

23. MedlinePlus, "Legionnaire's Disease," www.nlm.nih.gov/medlineplus/eny/article/000616.htm (accessed October 18, 2010).

24. Health Canada, "Bacterial Waterborne Pathogens. Current and Emerging Organisms of Concern: Legionella," January 7, 2008, www.hc-sc.gc.ca/ewh-semt/pubs/water-eau/pathogens-pathogenes/legionella-eng.php (accessed October 18, 2010).

Chapter 4

1. National Institute of Allergy and Infectious Disease, "Pneumococcal Pneumonia: Prevention," www.niaid.nih./gov/topics/pneumonia/pages/prevention.aspx (accessed November 1, 2010).

2. Stupka, "Community-Acquired Pneumonia in Elderly Patients."

3. M. L. Jackson, et al., "The Burden of Community-Acquired Pneumonia in Seniors: Results of a Population-Based Study," *Clinical Infectious Diseases* 39, no. 11 (2004): 1,642–1,650.

4. Genetics Home Reference, "Common Variable Immune Deficiency," March 2010, ghr.nlm.nih.gov/condition/common-variable-immune-deficiency (accessed October 19, 2010).

5. Tessa Wardlaw, et al., *Pneumonia: The Forgotten Killer of Children* (Geneva, Switzerland: World Health Organization, 2006).

6. John-Michael, Gamble, et al., "Admission Hypoglycemia and Increased

Mortality in Patients Hospitalized with Pneumonia," *American Journal of Medicine* 123, no. 6 (June 2010): 556.e11–556.e16.

7. Sarah D. Berry, et al., "Survival of Aged Nursing Home Residents with Hip Fracture," *Journal of Gerontology: Series A* 64A, no. 7 (July 2009): 771–777.

8. Samantha F. Ehrlich, et al., "Patients Diagnosed with Diabetes Are at Increased Risk for Asthma, Chronic Obstructive Pulmonary Disease, Pulmonary Fibrosis, and Pneumonia but Not Lung Cancer," *Diabetes Care* 33, no. 1 (2010): 55–60.

9. Shoshana J. Herzig, et al., "Acid-Suppressive Medication Use and the Risk for Hospital-Acquired Pneumonia," *Journal of the American Medical Association* 301, no. 20 (2009): 2,120–2,128.

Chapter 5

1. National Institute of Allergy and Infectious Diseases, "Pneumococcal Pneumonia: Complications," January 30, 2006, www.naid.nih.gov/topics/pneumonia/Pages/complicatons.aspx (accessed November 8, 2010).

2. Centers for Disease Control and Prevention, National Center for Immunization and Respiratory Diseases, "Pneumococcal Diseases and Pneumococcal Vaccines," May 2009, www.cdc.gov/vaccines/pubs/pinkbook/downloads/Slides/Pneumo11.ppt (accessed October 27, 2010).

3. J. H. Flory, et al., "Socioeconomic Risk Factors for Bacteremic Pneumococcal Pneumonia in Adults," *Epidemiology and Infection* 137, no. 5 (2009): 717–726.

4. Hui Yu, et al., "Lung Abscess Caused by *Legionella* Species: Implication of the Immune Status of Hosts," *Internal Medicine* 48 (2009): 1,997–2,002.

5. José da Silva Moreira, et al., "Lung Abscess: Analysis of 252 Consecutive Cases Diagnosed between 1968 and 2004," *Jornal Brasileiro de Pneumologia* 32, no. 2 (2006): 136–143.

6. D. G. Ashbaugh, et al., "Acute Respiratory Distress in Adults," *Lancet* 2 (1967): 319–323.

7. MedlinePlus, "Acute Respiratory Distress Syndrome," January 22, 2010, www.nlm.nih.gov/medlineplus/ency/article/000103.htm (accessed October 22, 2010).

8. National Heart, Lung, and Blood Institute, "ARDS: Key Points," www.nhlbi.nih.gov/health/dci/Diseases/Ards/Ards_Summary.html (accessed October 22, 2010).

9. MedlinePlus, "Empyema," National Institutes of Health, March 17, 2009, www.nlm.nih.gov/medlineplus/ency/article/000123.htm (accessed November 1, 2010).

10. Joanne M. Langley, et al., "Empyema Associated with Community-Acquired Pneumonia: A Pediatric Investigator's Collaborative Network on Infections in Canada (PICNIC) Study," *BMC Infectious Diseases* 8 (2008), www.biomedcentral.com/1471–2334/8/129 (accessed October 29, 2010).

11. Pilishvili, "Pneumococcal Disease."

12. Cunha, *Pneumonia Essentials.*

13. Paul Ellis Marik, *Handbook of Evidence-Based Critical Care*, 2nd ed. (New York: Springer, 2010).

14. Michael C. Reade, et al., "The Prevalence of Anemia and Its Association with 90-Day Mortality in Hospitalized Community-Acquired Pneumonia," *BMC Pulmonary Medicine* 10 (March 16, 2010), www.biomedcentral.com/1471–2466/10/15 (accessed October 19, 2010).

15. Laura M. Cecere, et al., "Long-Term Survival After Hospitalization for Community-Acquired and Healthcare-Associated Pneumonia," *Respiration* 79 (2010): 128–136.

16. Scott T. Micek, et al., "Health Care-Associated Pneumonia and Community-Acquired Pneumonia: A Single-Center Experience," *Antimicrobial Agents and Chemotherapy* 51, no. 10 (2007): 3568–3573.

17. Maraya D. Zilberberg, et al., "Antimicrobial Therapy Escalation and Hospital Mortality Among Patients with Health-Care–Associated Pneumonia: A

Single-Center Experience," *Chest* 134, no. 5 (November 2008): 963–968.

Chapter 6

1. Marik, *Handbook of Evidence-Based Critical Care.*
2. Marre, "Detection of Respiratory Bacterial Pathogens."
3. H. Kothe, et al., "Outcome of Community-Acquired Pneumonia: Influence of Age, Residence Status and Antimicrobial Treatment," *European Respiratory Journal* 32, no. 1 (July 2008): 139–146.
4. Medscape, "Streptococcus Pneumoniae: Epidemiology and Risk Factors," www .medscape.com/viewarticle/521337_print (accessed September 24, 2010).
5. Mandell, "Consensus Guidelines."
6. Steven Schmitt, "Community Acquired Pneumonia," Cleveland Clinic Center for Continuing Education, August 1, 2010, www.clevelandclinicmeded.com/ medicalpubs/diseasemanagement/ infectious-disease/community-acquired-pneumonia (accessed January 9, 2011).
7. Mandell, "Consensus Guidelines."
8. Marik, *Handbook of Evidence-Based Critical Care.*
9. Marre, "Detection of Respiratory Bacterial Pathogens."
10. Mandell, "Consensus Guidelines."
11. Serpil Ercis, et al., "Validation of Urinary Antigen Test for *Streptococcus pneumoniae* in Patients with Pneumococcal Pneumonia," *Japanese Journal of Infectious Diseases* 59, no. 6 (2006): 388–390.
12. Mark H. Ebell, "Outpatient vs. Inpatient Treatment of Community-Acquired Pneumonia," *Family Practice Management* 14, no. 4 (April 2006): 41–44.
13. Colleen R. Zaccard, Richard F. Schell, and Carol A. Spiegel, "Efficacy of Bilateral Bronchoalveolar Lavage for Diagnosis of Ventilator-Associated Pneumonia," *Journal of Clinical Microbiology* 47, no. 9 (September 2009): 2,918–2,924.
14. Centers for Disease Control and Prevention, "Antiviral Drugs for Seasonal Flu," December 22, 2010, at http://www.cdc .gov/flu/about/qa/antiviral.htm (accessed January 20, 2011).

15. Centers for Disease Control and Prevention, National Center for Immunization and Respiratory Diseases, "What You Should Know About Flu Antiviral Drugs," www.cdc.gov/flu/pdf/antiviral_factsheet 1011.pdf (accessed October 29, 2010).
16. Harvey Simon, and David Zieve, University of Maryland Medical Center, "Pneumonia-Medications," March 29, 2009, www.umm.edu/patiented/articles/ what_antibiotics_used_pneumonia_ 000064_8.htm (accessed November 8, 2010).
17. Centers for Disease Control and Prevention, "Antiviral Drugs for Seasonal Flu," www.cdc.gov/flu/about/qa/antiviral.htm (accessed November 20, 2010).
18. Centers for Disease Control and Prevention, "Invasive Pneumococcal Disease in Children 5 Years after Conjugate Vaccine Introduction—Eight States, 1998–2005," *Morbidity and Mortality Weekly Report* 57 (2008): 144–148.
19. Centers for Disease Control and Prevention, "People at High Risk of Developing Flu-Related Complications," September 3, 2010, www.cdc.gov/flu/about/disease/ high_risk.htm (accessed October 22, 2010).
20. Centers for Disease Control and Prevention, "Self-reported Influenza Vaccination Coverage Trends 1989–2008 among Adults by Age Group, Risk Group, Race/Ethnicity, Health-Care Worker Status, and Pregnancy Status, United States, National Health Interview Survey (NHIS)," www.cdc.gov/ flu/professionals/vaccination/pdf/ NHIS89_08fluvaxtrendtab.pdf (accessed November 19, 2010).
21. Centers for Disease Control and Prevention, "Pneumococcal Disease."
22. Gold and Adamec, *The Encyclopedia of Alcoholism and Alcohol Abuse.*
23. Spellberg, "Antibiotic Resistance."
24. GAVI Alliance, "The Gambia Introduces Vaccine Against World's Leading Vaccine-Preventable Child Killer," www.gavialliance.org/media_centre/ press_releases/2009_08_19_gambia_ pneumococcal.php (accessed November 20, 2010).

acute respiratory distress syndrome (ARDS) —A very serious complication of pneumonia that can lead to permanent lung damage or death.

antibiotic-resistant pneumonia—A form of pneumonia that does not respond to conventional antibiotics. Methicillin-resistant *Staphylococcus aureus* (MRSA) is an example.

antibiotics—Medications that are administered to kill bacteria.

antivirals—Drugs that combat viral infections in the early stages of disease.

bacteremia—Bacteria that is present in the bloodstream and can be identified with a blood culture.

blood culture—Using a sample of the patient's blood to grow bacteria in the microbiology lab.

bronchial pneumonia—Pneumonia that affects both lungs. Sometimes called double pneumonia.

community-acquired pneumonia—Pneumonia that is contracted when a person is not hospitalized or living in a nursing home.

dyspnea—Shortness of breath, a common symptom occurring among individuals who have pneumonia.

empyema—The presence of infected fluid in the area between the lung and the chest wall; a very serious medical condition.

Gram's stain—A laboratory test that shows the type of bacteria that infects the person with pneumonia by the color and shape of the pathogens. Gram-positive microbes present as blue or violet with this test, while gram-negative bacteria show as pink or red.

health care–associated pneumonia—Pneumonia caused by pathogens that the individual picked up while in a health care setting, such as while receiving dialysis treatments, cancer care, or other types of treatments.

hospital-acquired pneumonia—Pneumonia that develops while an individual is hospitalized for another medical problem.

human immunodeficiency virus (HIV) —A virus that is contracted through sexual contact with an infected person or through shared needles among those injecting illegal drugs. Infants born to infected mothers may contract HIV. This virus suppresses the immune system of infected individuals.

influenza (flu)—A viral infection that can lead to the development of pneumonia.

invasive pneumococcal disease (IPD) —Pneumonia, bacteremia, or meningitis that is caused by *Streptococcus pneumonia* bacteria. It is a leading cause of death in the elderly.

Legionella—A pathogen that can cause severe and even fatal pneumonia. Usually contracted from contaminated water.

lung abscess—A pus-filled cavity of the lung that is usually caused by the bacteria that also cause pneumonia.

nosocomial pneumonia—A term sometimes used to denote hospital acquired pneumonia.

pulse oximetry—The use of a noninvasive device that measures the level of oxygen in the blood. This is important in patients with pneumonia because if their oxygen level drops, they need supplemental oxygen in order to breathe.

sepsis—A condition of severe inflammation in response to infection that is a life-threatening condition. It can be a complication of pneumonia.

sputum—The material that is coughed up from the lungs by a patient with pneumonia or other lung diseases.

Streptococcus pneumoniae—A bacteria that frequently causes pneumonia, especially community-acquired pneumonia. Also known as *pneumococcus*. It can also cause infections and meningitis.

urinary antigen test—A test that measures antigens in the urine and that can rapidly determine if pneumonia-causing bacteria are present as well as identify the bacterium.

ventilator-associated pneumonia—Pneumonia that develops in a patient who is breathing with a mechanical ventilator.

Books and Articles

Burke A. Cunha, M.D., *Pneumonia Essentials,* 3d ed. Boston: Jones and Bartlett Publishers, 2010

Centers for Disease Control and Prevention. "Pneumococcal Disease." Available online at www.cdc.gov/vaccines/pubs/pink book/downloads/pneumo.pdf. Accessed on November 12, 2010.

National Heart, Lung, and Blood Institute. "What Causes Pneumonia." Available online at www.nhlbi.nih.gov/health/cdi/ Diseases/pnu/pnu_causes.html. Accessed October 22, 2010.

National Institute of Allergy and Infectious Disease. "Pneumococcal Pneumonia: Prevention." Available online at www.niaid.nih ./gov/topics/pneumonia/pages/prevention.aspx. Accessed November 1, 2010.

Web Sites

American Lung Association
http://www.lungusa.org

American Thoracic Society
http://www.thoracic.org

Centers for Disease Control and Prevention
http://www.cdc.gov

Food and Drug Administration
http://www.fda.gov

Immune Deficiency Foundation
http://primaryimmune.org

Immunization Action Coalition
http://www.immunize.org

Infectious Diseases Society of America
http://www.issociety.org

National Foundation for Infectious Diseases
http://www.nfid.org

National Heart, Lung, and Blood Institute
http://www.nhlbi.nih.gov

National Institute of Allergy and Infectious Diseases
http://www.niaid.nih.gov

World Health Organization
http://www.who.int

Christine Adamec has authored and coauthored many books for Facts On File, including *The Encyclopedia of Alcoholism and Alcohol Abuse* (2010), *The Encyclopedia of Drug Abuse* (2008), *The Encyclopedia of Elder Care* (2009), *The Encyclopedia of Phobias, Fears, and Anxieties* (2008), *The Encyclopedia of Child Abuse*, third edition (2007), and numerous other titles on pivotal medical and psychological issues. In addition, Adamec authored *Pathological Gambling* (2010) for Chelsea House's Psychological Disorders series.

Hilary Babcock, M.D., M.P.H., is an assistant professor of medicine at Washington University School of Medicine and the medical director of occupational health for Barnes-Jewish Hospital and St. Louis Children's Hospital. She received her undergraduate degree from Brown University and her M.D. from the University of Texas Southwestern Medical Center at Dallas. After completing her residency, chief residency, and infectious disease fellowship at Barnes-Jewish Hospital, she joined the faculty of the infectious disease division. She completed an M.P.H. in public health from St. Louis University School of Public Health in 2006. She has lectured, taught, and written extensively about infectious diseases, their treatment, and their prevention. She is a member of numerous medical associations and is board certified in infectious disease. She lives in St. Louis, Missouri.